108 Yoga and Self-Care Practices for Busy Mamas

Julie M. Gentile

For information, contact
MSI Press
1760-F Airline Highway, #203
Hollister, CA 95023

Photos © Copyright by Laura Brown Photography

Cover design and layout by Carl Leaver

Copyediting by Mary Ann Raemisch

LCCN: 2018968235

ISBN: 978-1-942891-84-0

This book is for informational purposes only and should not be used as a substitute for professional medical advice, diagnosis, or treatment. Speak with your doctor before beginning any new exercise routine.

To mamas everywhere: Shine the light on your own self-care so you can help lead the next generation—and the world—to wellness.

"Julie M. Gentile's experience as a parent of two young children, marketing and communications professional, and yoga teacher qualifies her as an ideal guide and inspiration for other moms trying to balance family, career, and their own self-care journey."

—Lori Gaspar, Founder and Director of Prairie Yoga

"Julie M. Gentile, a beautiful spirit, a warm, compassionate soul, continues to educate the community about yoga, encouraging others to find balance and peace within. The courage she has in taking the next step to write her book is nothing short of amazing. So powerfully inspiring."

—Christy Studant, Ayurvedic Practitioner, Founder/Co-owner of Mindful Movements and Owner of Live Powerfully

"Julie M. Gentile totally gets today's busy moms and has written a book that makes it super easy for them to finally put their needs at the top of their long to-do lists. Julie has been a mom advocate since the days she interned at Chicago Parent, and now that she is a mom herself, she's able to put that passion, drive, and knowledge to good use."

—Tamara L. O'Shaughnessy, Editor and Associate Publisher of Chicago Parent

Contents

Gratitude and Acknowledgments

I hold deep gratitude in my heart for all of the yoga teachers, mama leaders, and wellness authors who have come before me and who have inspired me to share my experience as a working mama, yoga teacher, and writer.

At the peak of my thank-you list is my talented and extraordinarily creative husband Mike Gentile—a dad, musician, writer, teacher, and leader. You light up my life. Thank you for supporting me on my self-care journey for more than half of our lives and for being the first reviewer of my first book. Your unique perspective as a busy dad adds sparkle and life force to my ideas! You have watched me dance with and seek balance along my wellness path, and you have witnessed first-hand the powerful force of self-love and how it can serve others. I am blessed to share my life with you. Thank you.

To my beautiful, sweet-hearted children, Vincent and Grace: I love all that you are and everything you will be. I look forward to guiding you as you walk your own self-care paths. May you find and come back to self-love at every turn along the way.

An abundance of deep gratitude for my own hard-working mama, Sue Liotine, who introduced me to my lifelong love of books and learning, and for my dad, Lou Liotine, for his dedication, perseverance, and mentorship, and for providing the groundwork to help me realize my greatest potential. To my gorgeous-spirited little sisters, Annie Liotine and Emilie Liotine, thank you for your listening ears and expansive, open hearts and minds. The Liotine family is a family of courageous leaders, and I am blessed to be a part of it.

An enormous thank you to my mama-in-law, Judy Gentile, and father-in-law, Nino Gentile, for watching my children while I work and work some more. Your love, generosity, and kindness is noted every day and will forever be appreciated.

To my extended Liotine family, Salerno family, Gentile family, O'Connor family, and Tyda family, and to my other dear family members and friends who aren't mentioned on these pages but who are always in my heart and on my mind, thank you for sharing your experiences and being a source of light and love.

A sincere thank you to the MSI Press team for the guidance, work, and dedication to helping me manifest this book.

Thank you to Laura Brown of Laura Brown Photography for the beautiful photos included on these pages and for your incredible imaging expertise.

Thank you to my students—on and off the mat—for serving as continuous inspiration.

To my readers, I am truly blessed and I am so very thankful for the opportunity to help guide you along your self-care journey by inspiring you to take impeccable care of yourself, even as busy as you are.

It is my ultimate hope that this book will inspire more moms to confidently become their own wellness leaders by actively prioritizing self-care so they can positively influence their families, friends, coworkers, and the world, and more fully enjoy their time on this beautiful earth.

Introduction

I wrote what you are about to read at the center of my very full life as a mom of two young children, working full-time as a marketing and communications professional, and leading yoga classes as a certified and registered yoga teacher. At that time, my husband was also working and going to school full time. "Full" is the key word here. With full hearts and full plates, we were bursting with busyness.

Many days pushed me beyond my limits, bringing me to tears of exhaustion and left me wondering if I was living life to my maximum potential. I was overcome with responsibilities that pulled me in multiple directions, but in me remained my ultimate duty to take care of myself. How did I do that as a working mama in an era where I was available via text message, phone, email, and social media?

I called upon my yoga and meditation background to help. It responded loud and clear: Take incredible care of yourself now so you can take care of the others in your life. Part of my ultimate wellness path is sharing what I've learned along the way with you, so you can easily transition from caring for others around the clock to caring more for you.

In observing and having conversations with others, I've found that there is opportunity for more people to take better care of themselves. They might eat nourishing meals, but they might not prioritize exercise or quality sleep. They might excel in their careers or be super-engaged parents, but self-care is low on their to-do list. Once taking care of yourself becomes your No. 1 priority, you will become a master of your own well-being. People will notice, and they will want that for themselves. Your ability to inspire others will be unstoppable.

As the author of numerous health and wellness articles, and taking what I have learned from a decade of practice on the four corners of my yoga mat, I have gathered inspiring tips and tools that I bring with me off my mat and onto these pages. These tools have served as a source of strength and steadiness for me, and they will help you persevere through your most chaotic moments as a mama, too.

It is an honor to serve as your personal wellness mentor as you set out to stand up for your self-care. I definitely get it—being a mama in the 21st century can be overwhelming. It's stop-what-you're-doing-right-now demanding. That's why I designed this book to help you be the best version of you in everything you do, and it starts with self-care. These pages ask you to take a close look at your self-care and mindfully explore how your mind, body, and soul can radiate with wellness.

Self-care is about taking care of your full being: mental, emotional, physical, spiritual, and beyond. It's taking time to pay attention and to determine what it is you need to live a vibrant, healthy, happy life where you get to decide what comes next. It is not acceptable to sacrifice your self-care in the face of busyness.

In this book, you will find 108 (a sacred number in yoga) writing prompts, yoga poses, meditations, breathing exercises, and other wellness practices to inspire you to walk a path of self-love. I've listed the practices that work for me, but this book is not an exhaustive list of self-care practices. This book was designed to help kick-start your self-care journey.

It is my wish for you that the following pages will spark an inner wellness revolution, help you build lifelong self-care practices, and serve as a dynamic guide so that you can realize your highest wellness potential and inspire that same transformation in others.

Drink from the fountain of wellness and delight in all that it has to offer. Take your time writing and reflecting, and take what you need from these pages. Own this experience. Make it yours. Then watch your wellness come to life.

I am excited to show you how to grow your self-love!

From my heart to each one of your hearts, namaste.
Julie M. Gentile

How to Use This Wellness Guide

This book was designed by a working mama to inspire other modern mamas to live well in this high-speed world. So many mothers are rushing through life, looking down at their phones, stressed, worried, anxious, pressed for time, and trying to do it all—to be a good mama, a good partner, a good employee, a good friend, and more. Too many mamas are sacrificing self-care. I lived this life, too. Something had to give, so I gave to myself. I took charge of my self-care and so can you.

In this book, each topic has a **Write about it** section, to record your thoughts, and a **Practice it** section, so you can practice a yoga pose or sequence, an Ayurvedic practice, meditation, a breathing exercise, or another wellness practice related to the topic in order to help you live a vibrant life. These beautiful, life-changing practices don't take time; they give you time. Discover how you can incorporate them into real life. Try them all. Continue the ones that resonate with you.

You've opened this book, so you're already halfway there to living a life devoted to self-care.

What you will need:

- a blank journal and a pen;
- a yoga mat (not necessary, but if you already own one, you can use it); and
- an open mind.

Where Should You Begin?

"Begin anywhere." —John Cage

I repeat this quote to myself daily, most often when I find myself immersed in a mountain of to-dos. These two simple words remind me that it's OK to start anywhere, from any direction. You can start this book from the beginning, work backwards, or flip to a section that calls to you right now. The important part is not where you begin your path to self-care, but that you start.

Significance of 108

The number 108, considered a sacred number in yoga, references spiritual completion. The number has a connection to nature and the cosmos. You'll hear about yogis practicing 108 rounds of sun salutations and reciting a mantra 108 times on a mala, a string of 108 prayer beads.

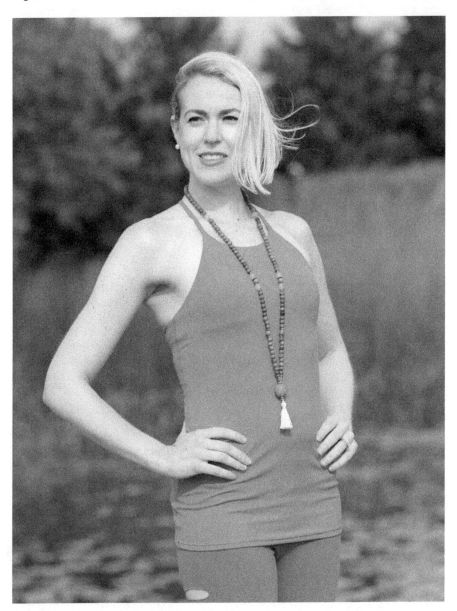

Set an Intention

At the beginning of each yoga class I lead, I ask students to set an intention for their practice. An intention—known as a *sankalpa* in Sanskrit (the language of yoga)—is a choice you make with your highest self. Dedicate an intention for yourself to help you walk this new path, the path of self-care and self-love. It can be as simple as learning something new about yourself or being open to making a necessary change to move you forward. With patience and practice, your intention will soon become a reality.

1   *Write about it: Dedicate an intention for your self-care journey*

Write your intention on a piece of paper and place it somewhere you will see it every day, such as your bathroom mirror or bedroom door.

2   *Practice it: Siddhasana (Accomplished Pose) with Hands in Anjali Mudra (Prayer Position)*

Seal your intention in your heart as you practice this quiet pose.

- Begin seated with your legs crossed, bringing one foot in front of the other. Ground your sit bones into the earth like the roots of a tree. Keep your spine tall and long. Relax your shoulders.

- Press your palms together at your heart, and allow your thumbs to connect with your heartbeat.

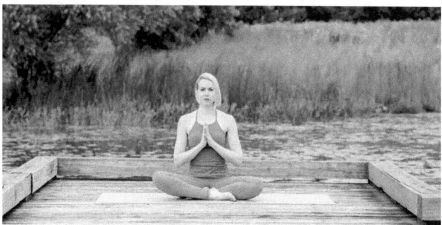

Siddhasana (Accomplished Pose) with Hands in
Anjali Mudra (Prayer Position)

What Brought You to This Wellness Guide?

I often ask my students what brought them to their mats. There is a reason they came to their practice, and there is a reason you picked up this book today.

3 *Write about it: Why do you care about self-care?*

See if you can connect your thoughts to the intention you set.

4 *Practice it: Urdhva Hastasana (Upward Salute)*

Offer your intention to the universe with this pose.

- Begin standing with your feet hip-distance apart.
- Sweep your arms to either side with your palms facing up and then overhead so your palms face each other. Gaze between your hands and feel the intensity of your intention.

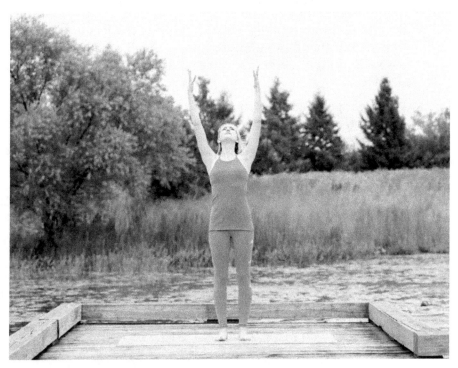

Urdhva Hastasana (Upward Salute)

Two Activities to Get You Started

"Whether you think you can, or you think
you can't, you're right." —Henry Ford

Embarking on a self-care path—a path dedicated to your wellness and longevity—is a sacred commitment to your well-being. It can be exciting and overwhelming. Know that your self-care journey and your intention won't look like anyone else's, which is what makes them absolutely beautiful.

5   *Write about it: Write where you need to be*

What are your wellness goals for the next month, year, and five years from now? Where are you now, and what are the steps you need to take to reach your potential?

6   *Practice it: Create a vision board and design a dedication space*

Vision Board

Take the next step to achieve your goals by creating a vision board, which is a visual representation of something in your life you are trying to manifest. The actual process of creating a vision board, which involves arranging inspiring images and words and pasting them to a poster board or paper, can help seal—and bring more clarity to—your intention.

I like to use my current intention as the theme of my vision boards. When I was newly pregnant with my daughter, I created a vision board for a healthy pregnancy. My board included several quotes, images, and words of encouragement, such as "Let the sun into your heart."

To get started on your own vision board, gather clippings from magazines, photos, inspiring quotes, and images aligned with your intention. Glue them on poster board in an arrangement that has meaning to you. Allow this beautiful creation to manifest into your truth. Display it in a spot you will see every day. Take a photo of your vision board and set it as the background on your smartphone or desktop to remind you of your intention.

Dedication Space

Create good vibes and keep your wellness inspiration flowing with a dedication space—an area in your home or office that includes a collection of meaningful items, such as photos, inspiring images, quotes, books, or objects that symbolize ideas you are cultivating in your life.

There are a few key items in my dedication space, but my space continues to evolve. My latest addition is a piece of rose quartz—a crystal with a soft pink hue—to help remind me to be more tender, loving, compassionate, and kind to myself.

Identify an area in your home or at work to display inspiring items. As new objects come into your life, add them to this space. A super simple way to start a dedication space is to display your vision board in that spot.

Practice Yoga Your Way

Yoga is officially everywhere these days—gyms, malls, parks, fitness centers, studios, schools, hospitals, offices, homes, and online. Its popularity has easily made it a $16 billion industry, and it will continue to grow as people get busier and more stressed. You probably know people who practice yoga, or you might already be a dedicated yogi.

The 2016 Yoga in America Study by Yoga Journal and the Yoga Alliance found that more than 36 million people in the U.S. practice yoga and almost three-fourths of those who come to their mats on a regular basis are women. And for good reason: 86 percent of yogis report having a strong sense of mental clarity, and 73 percent report being physically strong.[1]

If you haven't tried yoga, now is the time. Among its incredibly lengthy list of benefits, yoga

- helps you to slow down so you can become more mindful and aware of the present moment and everything that is arising in it—your thoughts, feelings, and sensations;

- serves as a top-notch stress reducer; and

- gives you an opportunity to put aside technology for a while and not have to respond to anybody but yourself—an unbelievable feeling.

Practicing yoga provides you with the resources and motivation to transform your spirit and your life in a magnificently uplifting way through *asana* (yoga poses), *pranayama* (breathing exercises), and *dhyana* (meditation). I cover several yoga poses, breathing exercises, and meditations in this book to get you started. These benefits don't just stop on your mat. You carry them right over into your daily life at home and at work, so really, everyone you encounter benefits from your practice.

There's good reason I refer to my yoga practice as my happy hour. Yoga has helped me restore and maintain health and vibrancy with joy, ease, and grace unlike anything else I have ever experienced. For a practice that originated more than 5,000 years ago, it still stands the test of time, and it is desperately needed in this fast-paced, modern world.

A decade ago, I had a miserable commute on a highway under construction. I needed a positive way to cope with my stress that didn't involve screaming, swearing, and beeping my horn in traffic. One day, I decided to try an evening yoga class after work. I didn't enter the class with any expectations other than I was hoping it would help me get a better handle on my stress.

It was so much more than that. It was mindful movement, learning how to breathe, and sitting with my thoughts, all in a beautifully blended package of a one-hour and 15-minute class. It provided me with a direct gateway to my inner peace—something I wasn't tapping into regularly. And it was fun! Before I walked out of class that night, I knew that I would lead yoga classes one day.

When I got home that night, I read my horoscope as I did every evening. It said that something new would enter my life that day and it referenced yoga. That's how fast yoga can work if you are open to it. Now I don't scream and swear at other drivers while in traffic.

7   *Write about it: Salute the essence of yoga within yourself*

List three ways you can realistically incorporate yoga into your weekly routine. For example, take a class, practice one yoga pose from this book every day, practice a 15-minute yoga sequence online, or all of the above.

8   *Practice it: Uttanasana (Standing Forward Fold)*

You don't have to wait until yoga class to start reaping the benefits of yoga. This pose is included in just about every yoga class. Try it to get an instant taste of self-care!

Standing Forward Fold is a gentle inversion that brings your head lower than your heart, helping to calm your mind, and reduce stress and anxiety.

- Stand with your feet hip-distance apart and your hands on your hips. Keep a soft bend in your knees, and from your hips, fold your upper body over your legs.

- Allow your hands or fingertips to touch the ground, your feet, or your legs. Keep your neck long so the crown of your head faces the ground.

- Stay here for three breaths. Then, when you're ready to come up, with a soft bend in your knees, allow your hands, arms, and head to remain heavy as you slowly roll up to standing, one vertebra at a time.

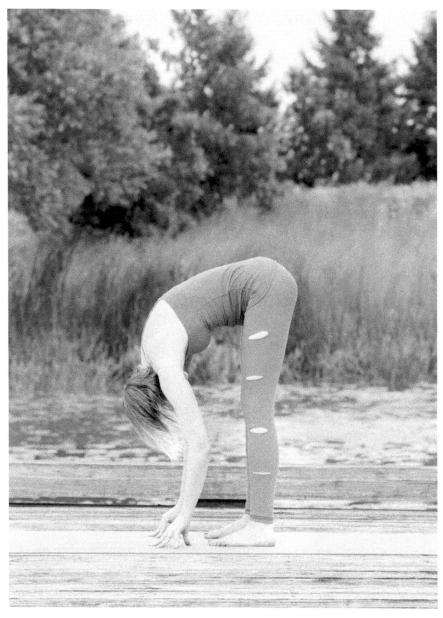

Uttanasana (Standing Forward Fold)

Julie M. Gentile

Make Life Better with Ayurveda

I fell deeply in love with self-care when I met Ayurveda. Ayurveda, the sister science of yoga, is one of the world's oldest medical traditions, which originated in India around the time yoga did. Ayurveda literally means the "science of life." It is a personalized approach to well-being and longevity that incorporates wellness rituals into everyday life. When paired with yoga, Ayurveda and yoga form an unmatched powerhouse.

I first learned about Ayurveda in my yoga teacher training in 2010, and that's when I started to experiment with Ayurvedic practices. Back then, I did not yet know how revolutionary these practices were until I began to weave them into my everyday life balancing a full workload as a working mama. Today, my everyday Ayurvedic practices include

- meditating, breathing exercises, and simple yoga stretches every morning, which typically take 10 to 20 minutes;
- following a consistent daily schedule of eating, working, and sleeping;
- oil pulling;
- drinking hot water with lemon throughout the day, which helps with digestion and detoxifies the liver;
- making lunch the largest meal of the day;
- eating mindfully (and not interacting with technology between bites);
- adding spices, such as turmeric, cumin, and ginger, to meals to help with digestion; and
- practicing abhyanga (self-massage with warm oil).

These are all simple things that I can realistically commit to practicing on a daily basis, but this is not a comprehensive list of all Ayurvedic practices. This book gives you a taste of what Ayurveda has to offer. The beauty of Ayurveda is that you have a lifetime to try all of the practices to find those that work best for you now and adjust your practices as you grow and evolve.

Ayurveda teaches that there are five elements found in the cosmic system: earth, water, air, fire, and ether (space). Everyone has a unique combination of these elements, which make up your mind-body type or *dosha*.

These combinations create three main doshas: vata (air and ether), pitta (fire and water) and kapha (earth and water). It is common to be dominant in one or two doshas. You were born with various amounts of each element, which make up your dosha at birth.

Leading a busy life can cause your doshas to become imbalanced. For example, your primary dosha when you were born may have been vata and your secondary dosha may have been pitta. Life as a modern mama may cause you to work too much, go to bed too late, and become more irritable, shifting your primary dosha.

Moving away from your original dosha can cause imbalances in your mind, body, and spirit. Once you get to know which dosha is dominant in your life now, you can choose specific Ayurvedic practices to help restore harmony to your well-being and get you back to your true nature.

One quick way to determine your dosha and discover Ayurvedic practices that can help you live vibrantly well is to take a dosha quiz online. These quizzes will ask you several health-related and lifestyle questions to help you identify your dosha.

You can take it a step further and schedule an appointment with an Ayurvedic practitioner (known as a *vaidya*) who is trained to create a customized lifestyle plan, based on your dosha and imbalances, to help restore you to optimum health.

9   *Write about it: Your dosha*

Take an online dosha quiz. Jot down whether the results are an accurate reflection of how you see your current health. What minor tweaks can you easily make for your well-being?

10 *Practice it: Oil pulling*

Oil pulling is an Ayurvedic practice to clean your mouth and pull out toxins by gently swishing oil around in your mouth. The more minutes you swish, the more benefits you receive. I typically swish sesame oil for a few minutes before I brush my teeth in the morning.

How to do it:

- Swish about one tablespoon of coconut oil or sesame oil (as long as you are not allergic to coconut or sesame) in your mouth for a few minutes, or as long as you can tolerate it up to 10 to 20 minutes. Swish the oil similar to how you would swish mouthwash.

- After you're done swishing, spit out the oil in the trash (not the sink!) since oil can clog your pipes. Also, you want to spit out the toxins, so don't swallow the oil you just swished.
- Brush your teeth.
- Enjoy the fresh feeling!

Meditate. Breathe. Repeat.

Meditation is magical. At first, I was hesitant to sit with scattered thoughts, but after attending many classes and workshops, meditation began to grow on me until it blossomed into a beautiful practice.

It isn't about completely clearing your mind of your thoughts. Meditation is sitting with your thoughts, without judging them, and noticing what feelings and sensations arise. Although traditionally practiced seated, you can meditate anywhere, any time. The more you meditate, the more you benefit. Reduced stress and anxiety, better concentration, and a better sense of clarity are just a few perks of a regular meditation practice.

Where does the magic come in? Meditation helps uncover your true self—your genuine wants, needs, hopes, and desires. If there is an important decision you need to make, meditate. If you're looking to find you're true calling in life, meditate. When you meditate, you create space for your spirit to speak.

As with yoga, there are many forms of meditation. I cover some of them in this book, so have fun exploring the different styles!

11 *Write about it: Your mind on meditation*

Record your thoughts about meditation—anything that comes to mind—and whether you think you can commit to a few minutes of meditation every day. Once you develop a regular practice, journal for a few minutes after each meditation about the themes and thoughts that came up during your session.

12 *Practice it: The one-minute meditation for modern mamas*

Practice this at home, at work, or anywhere you can. Set a timer with a gentle sound on your phone if you'd like.

- Begin in a comfortable seated position. Allow your spine to be tall and long. Relax your shoulders, and rest your hands on your knees or press your palms together at your heart. Gently close your eyes.

- Imagine a thin string lifting the crown of your head toward the sky.

- Bring your attention to your breath. Watch your inhales and exhales come and go. As thoughts enter your mind, acknowledge them and then watch them fade.

- Stay present. When the timer goes off, open your eyes.

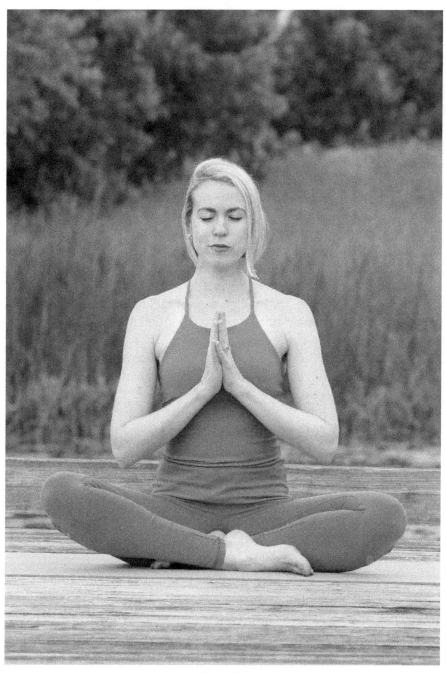

Seated Meditation

Calm Chaos by Being Mindful and Present

A few days before giving birth to my second child, my husband, my then 2-year-old son, and I went to a car dealership to see if we could trade in my husband's car for a van. It was wintertime, and my son was bundled up. We placed his car seat, with him in it, in the back seat of the van to test its fit. He whined and squirmed, and I knew something was up. His bedtime was approaching, and my husband was growing irritated. He wanted a few moments to ask the car dealer some questions. I gave my son a snack, and he quieted down. Then the whining started again, and he started to cough forcefully.

My mama intuition knew what was coming.

He vomited everywhere—all over his car seat, his coat, and the van, which we didn't yet own. After going through all of the wipes in his diaper bag, there was still more to clean. So there I was, nine months pregnant, walking back and forth into the car dealership bathroom to get paper towels (which eventually ran out) and toilet paper to clean up puke. But I wasn't frustrated. I continued to breathe slowly and steadily. After cleaning up the best we could, we left the dealership without the van.

A couple of days later, my husband went back to the same car dealership and traded his car for that van. When I look back on that experience, I see that I was practicing mindfulness. I maintained steadiness and calmness for my growing baby, my toddler, my husband, and myself. In the grand scheme of things, my son vomiting all over the van wasn't a big deal. Kids throw up. You wipe it up and move on.

Mindfulness doesn't just happen on a yoga mat. For many, that's where it starts, but it's off the mat and in real life (where you spend most of your time) where it is truly valuable. It's a centered way to calm everyday chaos.

In any given moment, if you observe your thoughts closely, most of them are about a past experience or a future event. When you're caught up in the busyness of life, it's easy to forget how to slow down and be present. Mindfulness helps you to live life more slowly and conscientiously in the present moment. It gets you back in touch with your senses and sensations in your body, and it helps you notice your thoughts, emotions, and feelings in every moment. It teaches you how to respond to situations instead of immediately reacting.

The mindfulness-based question I find myself asking most often is: *How can I embody my highest self in this moment?* With time and practice, mindfulness allows you to make decisions with your highest self, which can help you respond calmly to whatever life brings you, even cleaning puke in a van with limited cleaning supplies when you're very pregnant.

The following practices can help you start implementing mindfulness in your life right now and manage moment-to-moment chaos.

13 *Write about it: Measure your mindfulness*

Create a three-column table and label the left-hand column "Past," the middle column "Present," and the right-hand column "Future." In the "Past" column, write down thoughts you are holding onto from the past. In the middle column, write down thoughts that are currently popping up. In the "Future" column, write down events that have not yet happened but that you keep thinking about.

As you look at your lists, know that you can choose mindfulness by bringing more awareness to the present moment. Thinking about past events won't change them, and worrying about the future won't alter it. How can you stay present and tend to what is right in front of you?

14 *Practice it: Scan your senses in two mindful minutes*

Get in tune with the present moment by paying attention with the following practice. You can set a timer for two minutes if you'd like.

- Begin where you are with your eyes closed.
- Bring your attention to your breath. Watch your inhales and exhales come and go. Notice if your breath is smooth and steady or rapid and erratic.
- As thoughts of the day and your to-do list enter your mind, observe them without judgement.
- Notice if you are holding onto any tension in your body. Notice the touch of your sit bones on the chair or the ground. Notice where your hands are resting.
- Notice the sounds around you. Do you hear birds chirping in the distance or the hum of your dishwasher?
- Notice the smells around you. Is something baking in the oven or do you smell freshly cut grass from a nearby open window?
- Notice if there is a taste in your mouth. Does your mouth feel dry or are you thirsty?

- Notice your eyelids softly covering your eyes and what colors you visualize with your eyes closed.
- If your mind wanders, gently guide it back to your breath. When two minutes have passed, open your eyes. Notice if you feel more aware in the present moment.

Salute Your Definition of Self-Care

Self-care is more than brushing your teeth and taking a shower. It's specific daily rituals that you do to reduce your stress, restore your vitality, enhance your overall wellness, and help you age gracefully. Self-care is the most important thing you can do to show yourself love—it's taking time to take ultimate care of yourself.

Instead of thinking self-care is just another task you have to squeeze into an already packed schedule, choose practices from this book that you look forward to and enjoy.

You're probably aware of the lifestyle habits in the following list that can move you away from self-care:

- relying on caffeine, especially coffee, to get you through the day;
- going to bed too late;
- sleeping in too late;
- not exercising;
- not drinking enough water;
- drinking excess alcohol;
- eating when you're not hungry or overeating; and/or
- ignoring your body's signals and urges, such as holding your need to pee.

15 *Write about it: How you currently take care of yourself*

Write down 10 ways you take care of yourself on a weekly basis. Five years ago, I would not have been able to list 10 things. Are you able to list 10 things you do for self-care? If not, allow this exercise to serve as a reminder for you to make your health and wellness your top priority.

16 *Practice it: Utkata Konasana (Goddess Pose)*

Embody your inner self-care goddess with this pose.

- Stand with your feet three to four feet apart. Turn both sets of toes so they point outward with your heels turned inward.

- Bend your knees so they are stacked above your ankles, and lower your hips so they are aligned with your knees. Allow your thighs to be parallel to the ground.

- Take your arms to a "T" position and bend your elbows so they are aligned with your shoulders. Allow your palms to face forward and spread your fingers wide. Inhale to lengthen your spine, and on an exhale, sink a little lower.

- Stay here for three breaths and then release.

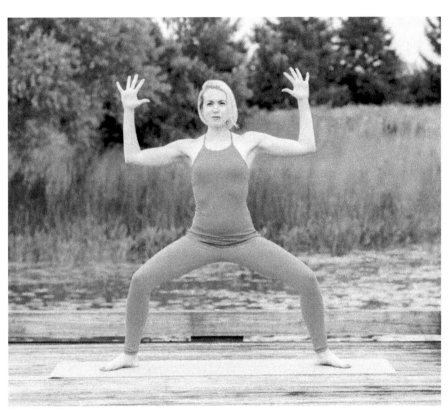

Utkata Konasana (Goddess Pose)

Identify Who You Are and What You Want

During my morning meditation, I often ask myself two questions: *Who am I and what do I want?* I don't need to immediately answer. Instead, I allow the questions to settle and provide space for the answers to come from my deepest self, which is always quietly and patiently waiting. As I go about my day at work or at home, I reconnect with these questions.

You are more than who you think you are—your personality, your job, your hobbies. There is only one beautiful you, and you have a unique gift. Are you ready to share it with the world?

17 *Write about it: Bring more meaning to this life*

Create a word cloud by writing words that make up *who you are* in one color. In a different color, write down *what you want*. In a third color, write down *how you can share your gifts* of who you are and what you want with the world in a meaningful way.

18 *Practice it: Observe your posture*

Your posture says a lot about who you are, such as where you hold stress and tension in your body and whether you present with confidence.

- Wherever you are right now, relax your shoulders and allow your spine to be tall and long.
- Stack your shoulders over your hips, and bring your inner ears over your shoulders, taking your head back in space slightly.
- Inhale and exhale deeply and observe how your body feels with these small tweaks to your alignment.

See Yourself More Clearly

Being your authentic self sounds easy, but in a world of judgement, it's not. Choices you make every day—how to raise your kids, how many hours to work, what to wear, how to cut your hair—set you up for judgment. Seeing yourself more clearly by naming your values, interests, passions, wants, and needs makes it easier to live the life you want to live, minimizing your attachment to what other people think.

19 *Write about it: The true you*

Write a crystal-clear description of your values, interests, passions, wants, and needs. Can you stay connected to the items on your list without being impacted by others' opinions?

20 *Practice it: Guided visualization meditation*

Guided visualization meditation can help you focus, center your breath, and tune in to your true self. When I first learned a version of the meditation below, I was brought to tears. With your eyes closed, ask someone to read the following meditation to you, and observe the emotions that awaken.

Imagine that you are walking alone on a beach on a late summer day. You've lost track of time, but you don't have any responsibilities today. You're well-rested and you've just had lunch, so you're perfectly content. The glowing sun touches your skin and instantly warms you from the outside in.

As you squish your feet into the sand with each mindful step, you notice that it feels slightly cool from the trace of the water that had been there only a moment before. You hear the gentle sound of a wave and feel the smooth water brushing up against your feet, washing the sand from them. As you gaze into the deep, steady sea, you pause for a moment, admiring the sun's reflection lighting up the water for what seems like miles.

The air smells pure and fresh. You lick your lips and taste the ocean. As you continue to walk further down the beach, the sound of a seagull overhead interrupts your thoughts.

You notice a hill with a stone path, and you are compelled to walk in that direction. As you walk up the cold stones, you see that there is someone sitting peacefully still at the top of the hill. You walk closer to get a better look. It is a woman, but she is facing the opposite direction. Her back looks familiar, so you take a few steps closer with the intention of greeting her. As you approach her side, you are overcome with a sense of familiarity, beauty, peace, and love. You walk a few more steps so that you are now standing directly in front of her.

Her energy and presence are breathtaking. You take a cleansing breath, and in that moment, you realize this woman is you. It is you sitting peacefully, calm, and centered.

You speak with her until the sun starts to set. You thank her and tell her you love her. As you walk away, you have a feeling of inner knowing, clarity, and contentment that everything is as it should be.

Honor What Excites Your Soul

A day full of responsibilities and expectations can be stressful and un-inspiring. What's one way to motivate you to get going? Identify your life's purpose. I wake with the intention to inspire others to live well every day, whether through my interactions with them, leading yoga classes, or writing. What do you live for? This single thing can motivate you more than the smell of coffee brewing.

21 *Write about it: What motivates you?*

Over the course of a week, ask yourself the following question as soon as you wake up: *What is motivating me to get out of bed?* Write down your answer every morning for seven days and see if this exercise can help you identify your life's mission.

22 *Practice it: Adho Mukha Svanasana (Downward-Facing Dog) and Plank Pose*

Strengthen your mind, body, and spirit and your commitment to what motivates you with this two-pose flow.

- Begin on your hands and knees in tabletop position with your hands slightly forward of your shoulders and your hips stacked over your knees. Spread your fingers wide.

- Curl your toes under as you straighten your legs and bring your sit bones toward the sky until your body is in an upside-down "V" position.

- Melt your heels toward the ground, and keep your head between your upper arms. Stay here for three breaths.

- Transition to Plank Pose by drawing your hips to the same level as your shoulders. Stack your heels over your toes. Allow your body to be in one long line from the crown of your head to your heels. Engage your abdominal muscles by hugging your belly button toward your spine.

- Stay here for three breaths. Flow between Plank Pose (on an inhale) and Downward-Facing Dog (on an exhale) a few times, and then release to your hands and knees in tabletop position.

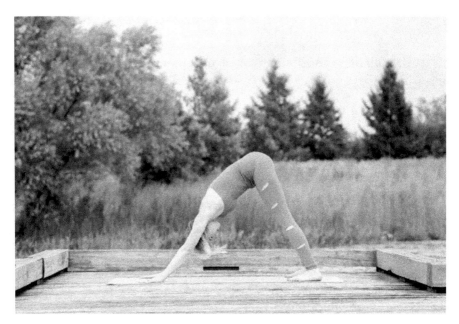

Adho Mukha Svanasana (Downward-Facing Dog)

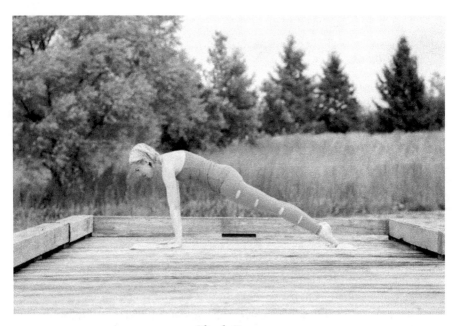

Plank Pose

Bring on Inner Bliss

It's 6 pm. You're deeply concentrating on reading a massive work email chain that requires your immediate attention, and you're next in line to respond. Your kids are getting restless because they need to eat dinner, take a bath, and go to bed. You haven't eaten or gone to the bathroom in hours. Suddenly, you have a flashback of playing in your childhood bedroom being a child again, enjoying the spaciousness of daydreaming and exploring. If everything but the daydreaming sounds like your average day, it's time to reconnect with your bliss.

When I was a child, I could sit for hours reading, writing, and making crafts. My favorite places to visit were libraries and bookstores. I didn't want toys. I wanted books. I have also always been eager to learn how to live well—from how much to exercise and what type of exercise to do to the healthiest foods to eat. When I started to take better care of myself, it was easier for me to reconnect with my true bliss, which I already knew when I was a child: to become an author and inspire others to live well.

23 *Write about it: Who did you want to be when you grew up?*

When you were a child, who did you say that you would become one day? Are you her today? If not, what's stopping you? What characteristics did you envision when you thought about the future you?

24 *Practice it: Sama Vritti (Equal Breathing)*

When your breath is still, so is your mind and body. I practice this breathing exercise when I want to get quiet. It helps ground me and reconnects me to my bliss.

You can practice this standing or seated, before you give a presentation, while sitting in traffic, or before you respond to your child's meltdown. The key is to match the length of your inhales and exhales.

- Seal your mouth slightly. Inhale through your nose to a count of four.

- Exhale through your nose to a count of four.

- Continue this pattern for several rounds and then come back to your natural breath.

Map Out Your Moments of Significance

There are moments in life that leave such an imprint on your heart that they are woven into your existence. These moments have the power to change the course of your life, and they serve as inspiring teaching tools. The following are some of my most memorable moments that have helped me grow on my journey.

- During the first yoga class I ever took, I felt an intense pull to become a yoga teacher.

- The moment I took my first step down the wedding aisle, an extraordinary sense of love washed over me, from the people in attendance to my husband, patiently waiting to call me his wife. As I walked closer to him, the gleaming light from the stained-glass windows grew brighter. I was filled with the warm glow of love and joy.

- I touched love in its purest form when I experienced the miraculous moments of my children entering the world. Hello, motherhood! Witnessing these new lives take their first breaths and snuggling with them for the first time, I was in awe of my body and the process of human creation. I remember thinking how courageous moms are, and how much incredible strength they have to grow a life for nine months, give birth, and then raise that child. I have so much respect for mamas everywhere.

- Within moments of my first-born child's birth, he needed to go to the neonatal intensive care unit (NICU), where he stayed to receive antibiotics for the first week of his life. My water had broken and I had been in labor for 24 hours. My son also initially had a weak cry (ironic because he now has a powerful voice). All of those things meant an admission to the NICU.

  I felt I had failed my son. I quietly cried during many of my new mama moments. My son was constantly being poked because he kept pulling out his intravenous line. I felt vulnerable and torn about my newborn being pumped with antibiotics, but I knew I had to be courageous. I would get him out of the NICU as fast as I could.

I questioned the doctor every day to see if there was a chance to get my son home earlier, but the answer was always the same. He needed the full course of antibiotics before he could be discharged.

During that week in the NICU, I learned how to be this beautiful boy's mama and how to breastfeed. Many new moms are discharged from the hospital before their milk comes in for the first time and need breastfeeding support as they learn how to feed their babies.

My son was discharged from the NICU when he was one week old. We went on to become a successful breastfeeding team for an entire year. The start to his new, precious life and to my motherhood was not what I had ever imagined, but I live in gratitude for this experience.

25 *Write about it: Moments that made an impact*

List the significant moments in your life. How have they altered the course of your existence?

26 *Practice it: Attend a yoga class today*

Practicing yoga can leave a significant imprint on your heart and enhance meaning in the moments that mean the most to you. There are dozens of styles of yoga—from chair yoga to vinyasa flow yoga to restorative yoga and more. You are bound to find something you like. My biggest tips for beginners (and more advanced practitioners, too) are

- to show up to class with an open mind;
- to listen to your body, which will help you stay safe; and
- to remain curious.

Even as a yoga teacher, I take classes weekly, and I attend workshops and trainings. Yoga is an ocean of knowledge, so take your time exploring its depth. It's called a practice for a reason. Little by little, you will evolve and transform your life.

Research a class at a local yoga studio or fitness center, rent DVDs from the library, or find yoga classes and videos online. As you become familiar with the poses, you can design a personalized sequence for your home practice.

Prioritize a Self-Care Day

There is no better treat than a moment to yourself, but what would you do if you had 24 hours to do anything you desired? I would meditate, practice yoga, get a massage, take a walk outdoors, journal, read an inspirational book, cook and eat nourishing foods, take a warm bath while sipping on tea, and go to bed early. And I wouldn't rush any of it; I would take my time.

27 *Write about it: Your ideal day*

If you were given a full day to do whatever you wanted, what would you do? Write a plan for your day of self-care. Once a month (or as often as you can), take a day where you can slow down, turn off your phone, and dedicate several hours to self-care.

If you can't commit to a whole day, set aside a couple of hours on a weekend where you won't be interrupted. Ask someone to watch your children, such as your partner or a relative, or hire a babysitter. Explain to that person the significance of this time for yourself. You owe it to yourself.

28 *Practice it: Marjaryasana-Bitilasana (Cat-Cow Pose)*

Treat yourself to these two simple poses daily. I practice Cat-Cow every morning because my spine craves it!

- Begin on your hands and knees in tabletop position with your shoulders stacked over your wrists and your hips stacked over your knees. Rest the tops of your feet on your mat or the ground.

- On an inhale, drop your belly toward the ground as you look up. Feel the stretch along the front of your belly. On an exhale, draw your belly button toward your spine as you round your upper back in a C-curve position.

- Continue to alternate between these two movements, using your breath as your guide. Inhale into Cow Pose and exhale into Cat Pose.

- Repeat up to 10 times.

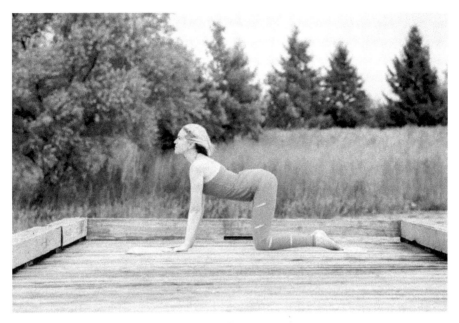

Bitilasana (Cow Pose)

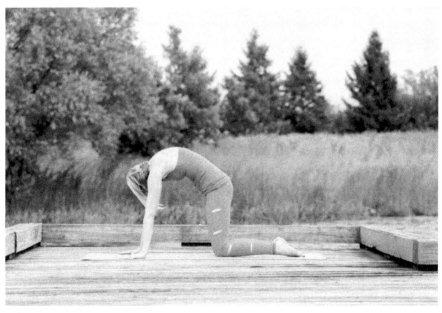

Marjaryasana (Cat Pose)

Ready, Set, Awaken! Start Your Day in a Powerful Way

"Each morning we are born again." —Buddha

This quote reminds me to start fresh every day. Each new day is a blank page of possibilities, and you get to write your story—beginning, middle, and end—for those 24 hours. How exciting!

Your typical morning routine might go something like this: You wake up to your alarm or to one of your kids talking or nudging you to get up. You turn over in bed and hit snooze because you're not ready to wake up. At the persistence of your children, you eventually force yourself to stumble out of bed and grab your coffee. At some point in between getting your kids ready for the day, you manage to get yourself ready.

You leave the house in a dash without eating breakfast, but that's OK— you grabbed a granola bar that you can gobble in the car on the way to work. You arrive late to drop off your child at preschool because he's curious about the bugs outside and the dew on the grass, which means you'll be late for work, too. Sound familiar?

Things can get pretty chaotic when you're trying to get yourself and your kids ready in the morning, so the last thing you want to do is spend more time on yourself when you just want to get out the door. You put off your own needs with a do-it-later mind-set, but when later comes, you might be too exhausted to find motivation for self-care. When you take a closer look at what you are actually doing in the morning (perhaps responding to emails and browsing social media is eating up your time), you might have more time for self-care than you think.

The way you begin your day sets the tone for the rest of it. Starting your day rushed will easily make you feel rushed and stressed throughout the day. You might have a feeling of not being able to catch up—responding to emails late, arriving late to meetings, picking up your kids late, going to bed late—and the cycle continues. On the flip side, starting your day calm, quiet, and inspired can help you maintain inner peace and steadiness throughout the day.

Ayurveda recommends that you start your day before the sun rises, when the earth is still and quiet. Rising before the sun can help you feel vibrant and refreshed. Waking after the sun rises can bring on a heavy, sluggish feeling.

I used to start my days with my fight-or-flight response kicked into high gear, rushing from one thing to the next. Once I realized that I have a choice in how I greet the morning, I began to make small tweaks.

Before I even leave my bedroom in the morning, I practice yoga, breathing exercises, and meditation for at least 10 minutes. On days I skip this routine, I notice a major difference in my energy, mood, and tolerance.

29 *Write about it: Wake up to inspiration*

Build a morning self-care plan that incorporates wellness practices you keep putting off. Use the ideas from this book to get you started. Keep tweaking your morning self-care routine until it feels good. You'll know it's working when it's easy for you to maintain a state of grace and ease throughout the day. Explore, experiment, and create a morning wellness blueprint no one has ever seen before.

30 *Practice it: Rise and shine yoga flow*

Practice this quick flow before a morning meditation or on its own.

- Begin standing with your feet hip-distance apart in Tadasana (Mountain Pose). Root your feet into the ground and equally distribute the weight in your feet.

- With your hands pressed together at your heart, take a deep inhale, and on the exhale, chant the sound *om* (which sounds like "home" without the "h" but traditionally pronounced *aum*) slowly. Repeat this two more times. The sacred sound of om is thought to be the first vibrational sound of the universe. If you've ever chanted om, especially in a group set-ting, you know its power.

- On an inhale, sweep your arms up overhead with your palms facing one another in Upward Salute.

- Exhale and sweep your arms to the sides and then down to Standing Forward Fold. Allow your hands or fingertips to touch the ground, your feet, or your legs. Relax your head and neck. Stay here for three breaths.

- Place your hands on either side of your feet and press your palms into your mat as you slightly bend your knees and step your feet back to Downward-Facing Dog.

- Keep your legs straight as you lift your sit bones toward the sky, melting your heels toward the ground. Stay here for three breaths.

- On an inhale, look at your hands, soften your knees, and as you exhale, mindfully walk your feet to meet your hands in Standing Forward Fold.

- On an inhale, soften your knees and allow your hands, arms, and head to get heavy. Slowly roll up one vertebra at a time so your head is the last thing to come up.

- Repeat this flow two more times. You're ready for whatever comes your way today!

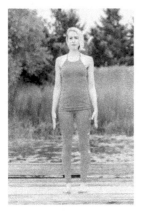

1) Tadasana
   (Mountain Pose)

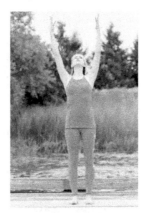

2) Urdhva Hastasana
   (Upward Salute)

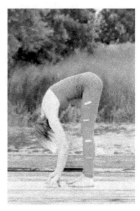

3) Uttanasana
   (Standing Forward Fold)

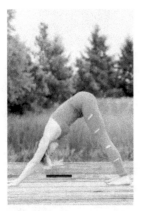

4) Adho Mukha Svanasana
   (Downward-Facing Dog)

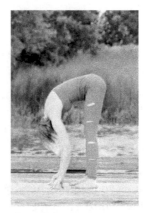

5) Uttanasana
   (Standing Forward Fold)

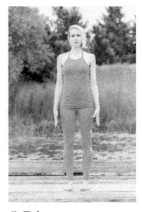

6) Tadasana
   (Mountain Pose)

Create a Routine You Love

A day in the life of a modern mama may mean non-stop driving, working, typing, talking, thinking, and rushing. Mealtimes, bath times, bedtimes, meetings, practices, appointments, trips to the store, and more mean that your schedule is full and different every day.

Your day is likely longer than anyone else's that you know, but your time is just as sacred as everyone else's time. Because you're so busy, every minute matters. In fact, you've probably been forced to become an expert in managing your time.

It's easy to get into the habit of saying "yes" to everything people ask of you, but that is a direct drain on your precious time and energy. Henry Ford said, "If you always do what you've always done, you'll always get what you've always got." If your current routine isn't working for you, tweak it until it does. If you don't, then you'll just keep repeating the same old story. Don't let the day slip away without spending time on yourself. Take action.

It helps to get organized by creating a realistic daily schedule that works for you and your family—and one that nourishes you enough to do it again tomorrow. In Ayurveda, *dinacharya*, which means daily routine, is one of the most powerful ways to find balance and boost your health. It involves eating, sleeping, and working at specific times and at about the same times every day—including weekends. Creating a daily rhythm brings your body into harmony (which your body really likes) as it learns to expect to eat, sleep, and work at consistent intervals.

There is no one specific schedule that works for everyone, but in general, Ayurvedic wisdom recommends that you

- wake up before the sun rises or around 6 a.m.;
- eat a warm, nourishing breakfast between 7 and 9 a.m.;
- work on your most important projects at work or at home between 10 a.m. and 2 p.m.;
- eat lunch—your largest meal of the day—between noon and 2 p.m. (when the sun and your digestive fire are at their fiercest);
- eat a small dinner between 5 and 7 p.m. (so you have time to digest your meal before bed and the digestion of your dinner doesn't interrupt your sleep);

- take it easy after dinner, practicing activities that help you turn inward, such as reading and journaling, to prepare your body for sleep;

- power down technology one to two hours before bed; and

- go to bed around 10 p.m.

31 *Write about it: Best times for you to eat, sleep, work, and practice self-care*

Using these Ayurvedic recommendations, list realistic times of the day for you to eat, sleep, work, and schedule self-care practices.

32 *Practice it: Test your new routine for a week*

Follow the schedule you created for seven days. At the end of the week, notice whether you were able to stick to it and how you felt. What still needs tweaking?

Rethink Your Work Week

The working world moves fast; does anyone actually feel caught up? In an environment where you're available by work phone, cell phone, email, and social media, it's easy to become overstimulated, overscheduled, overwhelmed, and overworked.

If you are a mama in the working world, you are likely highly efficient at making things happen and accomplishing multiple tasks and projects every day, so you do more. You may have become used to the continuously flowing emails and deadlines, and running from meeting to meeting without a break. You also likely place more demands and pressure on yourself than anyone else. Can you realistically sustain this way of living?

Think about when your stress levels are highest. It can be on your way to work, during work meetings, or a general feeling of being overwhelmed that you get from taking on too much. How can you minimize stress at work and make your current situation better? The first step is to set boundaries at work. Define the number of hours and times you'd like to work. Then look at other ways to weave in wellness into your workday, such as taking a lunch break every day or going for an afternoon walk outside.

33 *Write about it: Your stress triggers*

When are you most stressed at work? List three adjustments you can easily make to your work routine so that it is more enjoyable.

34 *Practice it: Six simple seated yoga stretches*

Imagine you're at work and it's mid-afternoon. Your bladder feels like it's going to burst, but you're trying to meet a deadline. Your phone rings and you see it is someone you have been waiting for to call you back. Do you answer it or do you dart to the bathroom? Modern mamas make these small decisions every day, and sometimes betray their own needs. What if you made the decision to be kinder to yourself at work?

Bring self-care with you to work with the following poses. Pick one pose or practice them all as a sequence whenever you have—or desperately need—a few moments to yourself.

Wrist Stretch

- Begin in a seated position. Relax your shoulders, and allow your spine to be tall and long.
- Stack your knees over your ankles. Allow the soles of your feet to rest on the ground.
- Extend your right arm in front of you as high as your heart with your palm facing forward and your fingertips facing up.
- Push your left hand into the fingers of your right hand to feel a stretch along your right wrist.
- After a few breaths, turn your right hand so your fingertips face down. Push your left hand into the fingers of your right hand to feel a stretch along your right wrist.
- After a few breaths, release. Repeat on the other side.

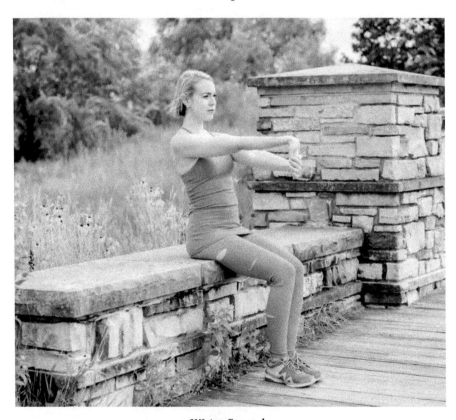

Wrist Stretch

Shoulder Relaxation and Rolls

- Relax your shoulders. Inhale both shoulders up to your ears. As you exhale, release them. Repeat three to five times.

- Make small forward circles with your shoulders a few times. Then gradually make the circles larger, moving slowly and mindfully. Repeat a few times, and then change directions.

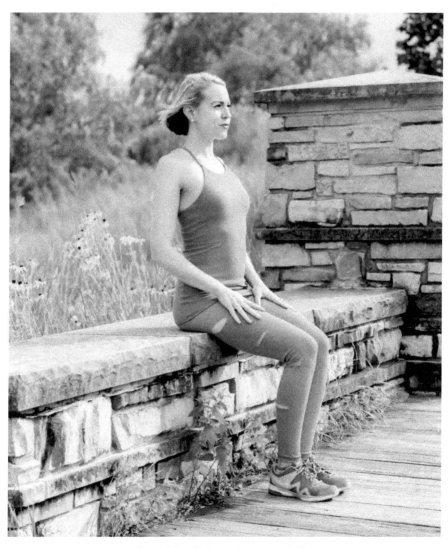

Shoulder Relaxation and Rolls

Garudasana (Eagle Pose) Arms, Variation

- Extend your arms out to a "T" position with your palms facing down. Cross your right arm over your left arm at your elbows. Bend your elbows and place your hands on your shoulders as if you're giving yourself a hug. Relax your shoulders.

- Stay here for a few breaths and then repeat on the other side.

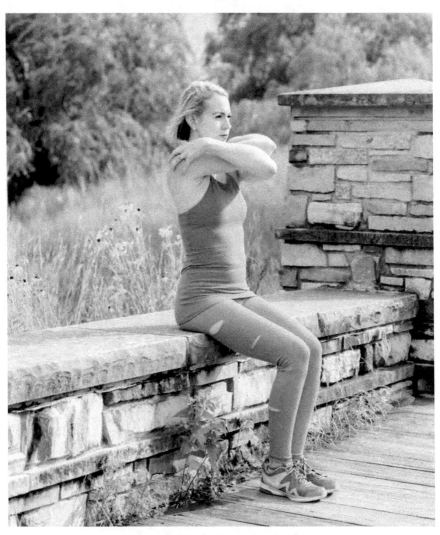

Garudasana (Eagle Pose) Arms, Variation

Seated Side Stretch

- Reach your arms overhead and interlace your fingers with your palms facing up. Relax your shoulders.
- Inhale, and on your exhale, stretch your arms and torso to your right side.
- After a few breaths, return to center. Repeat on the other side.

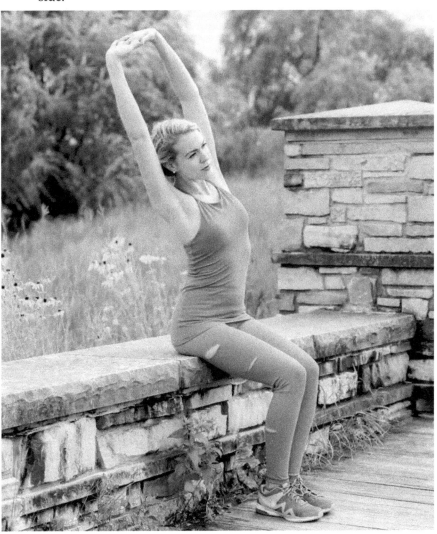

Seated Side Stretch

Seated Twist

- Place your right hand behind you, and place your left hand on the outside of your right knee or thigh.
- Inhale and allow your spine to lengthen, and as you exhale, twist to the right. Look over your right shoulder.
- After a few breaths, return to center. Repeat on the other side.

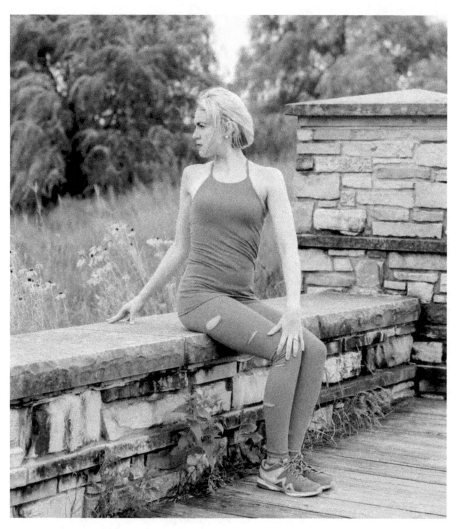

Seated Twist

Hip Stretch

- Begin with the soles of your feet rooted into the earth.
- Place the outside of your right ankle on top of your left thigh. Using your hands, place gentle pressure on the inside of your right thigh. Lean forward into the stretch.
- After a few breaths, switch legs.

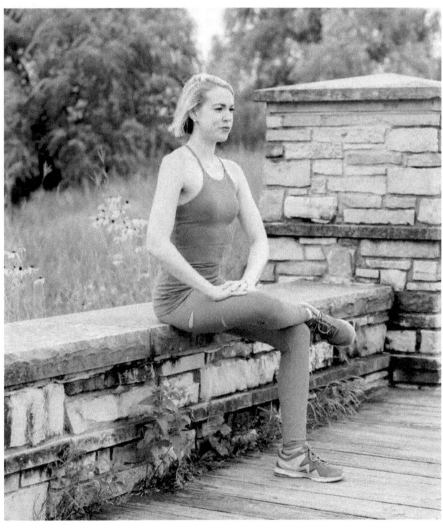

Hip Strech

Free Up More Me Time

In the age of hashtags and tagging, many hours of the day are devoted to technology. After the kids are in bed—a.k.a. prime "me" time—you might scroll through social media with the best intentions of limiting yourself to looking through posts for only a couple of minutes. Before you know it, two hours have gone by, and you're looking at a photo of someone you went to high school with posing at her cousin's wedding, wondering how you ever got there. Now the opportunity to spend those hours on yourself has passed.

It's not your fault.

You're used to being busy, so when you do get downtime, it can be difficult to know how to spend it. There is so much you can be doing. There are lunches to pack, emails to check, and news feeds to scroll through.

Stop giving away your precious free time to everyone (and everything) but yourself.

It's easy to watch TV and be drawn into the constant stream of stimulation on your smartphone, but this is distracted living. Distractions rob you of precious self-care. They separate you from how you really want to spend your time and lead to procrastination. What helps tune out distractions? Practice and discipline. Staying committed to your self-care will help you make decisions on how to spend your time.

35 *Write about it: How much of your day do you spend on yourself?*

When I first completed the following list of items, I gained clarity about the distractions that were withering away my self-care time.

On a daily basis, estimate the amount of time you spend (outside of work) on

- your smartphone (checking it, texting, making phone calls, and reading and watching online content);
- your computer;
- watching TV; and
- other electronic devices.

Add up the total number of hours. Out of these hours, how much time can you give back to self-care?

36 *Practice it: Detox from technology*

Choose a day off every week (if you work Monday through Friday, it can be a weekend day) to commit to a technology detox. Set your phone on airplane mode or switch it to silent and turn off email. If you can't be away from your devices for a full day, unplug for a few hours every weekend. Notice how you spend your time without technology.

Do Less

Until I began to respect my boundaries, I regularly pushed myself beyond my limits. Even though I knew better, I would push myself to work longer hours and stay up late to get more done. This way of living worked for a while, but over time, it depleted me. This is still a practice for me today, but I find that I say "no" more often to create space for self-care.

37 *Write about it: Shorten your to-do list*

This exercise will show you the big picture of all you do in a day. Create two columns. On the left, list your daily activities (e.g., getting ready for work, dinnertime); on the right, list the amount of time you dedicate to each activity. Can you remove or modify any activities, or replace them with self-care?

38 *Practice it: Jathara Parivartanasana (Revolved Abdomen Pose)*

This simple twist gently massages your internal organs. As with other twists, it also helps with digestion and elimination of foods, emotions, thoughts, and experiences.

- Begin by lying on your back.
- Bring your knees toward your chest and relax your arms in a "T" position at shoulder level on the ground with your palms facing up.
- Engage your abdominal muscles, and with your knees still bent, gently lower your legs to the right until they reach the ground. Keep your left knee stacked on top of your right knee. Melt both shoulders into the ground.
- To deepen the twist, take your right hand to the outside of your left knee and allow your head to turn to the left.
- After several breaths, bring your head and knees back to center. Repeat on the other side.

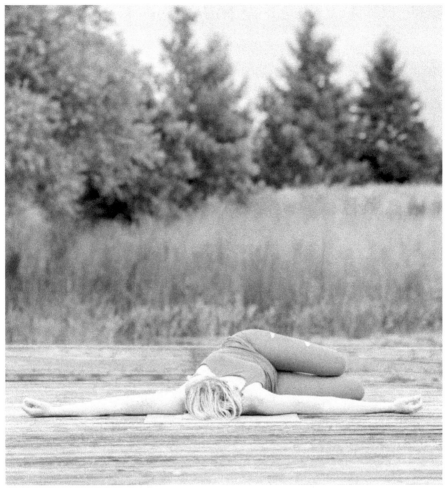

Jathara Parivartanasana (Revolved Abdomen Pose)

Ask for More Help More Often

I was standing in a long checkout line at the grocery store one afternoon, sweating because my then 2-year-old son was having a full-body meltdown on the floor. He missed his nap, and my baby was crying because she wanted to eat. As I stumbled to find my credit card in my wallet, the people behind us in line were mumbling under their breath and rolling their eyes. In that moment, I realized I needed help when taking two little ones to the store.

I don't need to do it all alone, and neither do you! Ask for help the next time you have to run errands. Recruit your partner, a family member, or a babysitter to watch your kids while you shop.

39 *Write about it: A call for help*

List everything you can think of that you can ask your partner, family members, coworkers, or friends to help you with at work or at home. It can be as simple as making a quick stop at the store or scheduling a meeting.

Remember to ask the universe for help, too. Is there something you want to invite into your life? Pose the question to the universe—write it down or meditate on it—and watch for the response, which may show up in unexpected ways.

40 *Practice it: Ananda Balasana (Happy Baby Pose)*

Babies need help to thrive. They let you know when they need something, such as milk, attention, or a snuggle, when they call out or cry. Give yourself attention by practicing this pose to channel your inner happy baby.

- Begin on your back, and draw your knees toward your chest.

- Separating your bent knees wider than your shoulders, extend both arms and place your hands on the outside of each foot or ankle, using your arms as resistance against your legs. Allow the soles of your feet to face the sky.

- Keep your back connected to the earth, or if it feels good, rock gently from side to side for a few breaths. Then release.

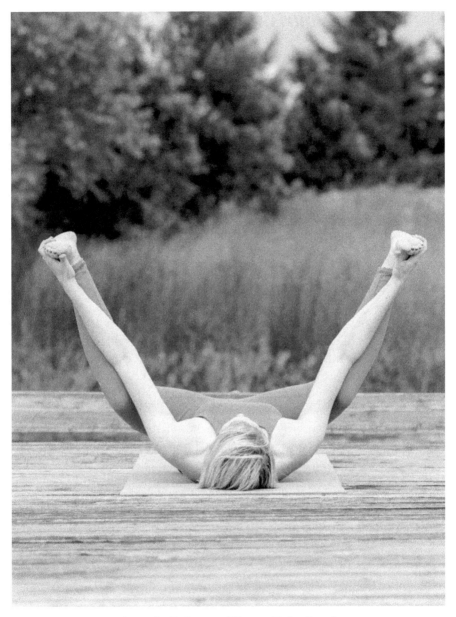

Ananda Balasana (Happy Baby Pose)

Nourish While You Eat

For several months, after most meals, I had extreme nausea and bloating. One day, I decided to investigate my symptoms.

After mindful observation, I learned that raw foods, such as carrot sticks, made me bloated, cold water made my stomach swell like a balloon, and too much gluten and dairy made me nauseous. Although I did not completely eliminate these foods, I slowly reduced them or changed the way I ate them. Instead of raw carrots, I ate cooked carrots. Instead of ice cold water, I drank warm or room temperature water. Little by little, I noticed a subtle difference. Like a thick fog dissipating, my nausea and bloating began to lift.

This first-hand experience solidified for me that food really does have the power to nourish or harm. The health of your body and mind are deeply impacted by the food choices you make. When you eat nourishing foods at the optimal times, your energy levels, mood, and immune system are more balanced.

Food is the building block for all of the systems in your body. Food contains *prana*, or life force. Plant foods, such as organic spinach and blueberries, are packed with prana. They grow from the earth and not in a factory. Processed foods, such as chips and crackers, don't contain a lot of prana.

Ayurveda teaches the importance of eating and cooking according to your dosha and the season to help make it easier for your digestive system to do its job. Look to nature and the season to help determine what to eat. For example, in the fall and winter, your inner environment can easily get cold, dry, and windy, just like the outdoors. If you eat cold, raw foods, like salad, in these seasons, it can cause constipation and bloating. However, eating warm, cooked, and slightly oiled foods, such as baked squash or apples in the fall and chicken soup in the winter, will help you feel your best.

Ayurveda also recommends that you

- cook with ghee (clarified butter);
- drink lots of room temperature water and warm water with lemon (which is used to help detoxify the liver and support digestion)—bloating be gone!;
- limit the leftovers you eat because they lack prana; and
- allow your digestive system to rest by not snacking between meals and not eating late at night, especially just before bed.

Where and how you eat matter, too. If you eat standing, in a rush, or while sitting in a car, your body's ability to digest your food well will be impacted. You might feel more bloated and sluggish after your meals if you don't allow yourself the time to sit, eat, and enjoy. At every meal, focus on the tastes and textures of your food instead of scrolling through your smartphone, watching TV, or working. Mindfully. Chew. Each. Bite.

41 *Write about it: Track your eating habits and mood for one week*

For seven days, record the times you ate, what you ate, where you ate, and how you felt after eating. What did you observe after keeping track of your eating habits for a week? How can you nourish yourself more at mealtimes?

42 *Practice it: Virasana (Hero Pose)*

In addition to it being a great stretch for your legs and ankles, Hero Pose can help you digest a meal when practiced right after eating.

- Kneel on the floor with the tops of your feet on the ground. If your knees need support, place a folded blanket under them.

- Touch your inner knees and thighs together but allow your feet to be slightly wider than your hips.

- Gently sit back toward the ground. If your sit bones do not touch the ground, rest them on a yoga block, book, or blanket. Let your spine be tall and long, and relax your shoulders.

- Place your hands on your thighs. Take several breaths.

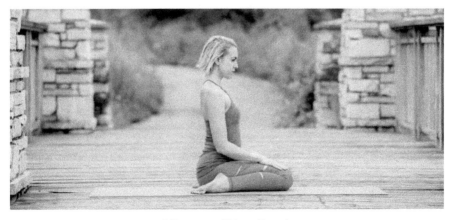

Virasana (Hero Pose)

Learn How to Make Nutrient-Dense Meals

Wild salmon, kale, garlic, quinoa, avocados, blueberries, almonds, eggs, turmeric, ginger, and dark chocolate, oh my! Do you incorporate these superfoods in your weekly meal rotation? My body craves all of these foods, but cooking doesn't come naturally to me. My husband is currently the main cook for our family. When I do cook, I follow recipes with precision. Learning how to prepare a variety of deeply nutritious meals is next up on my self-care journey. My mantra is to make every bite nutritious and make it fun.

43 *Write about it: Are you a natural in the kitchen?*

Do you love cooking or do you resist it? If you're not comfortable in the kitchen, list the things that would get you more interested in cooking.

44 *Practice it: Take a cooking class*

Give yourself the gift of a cooking class (or ask someone to pay the fee for the class as a gift for you). If you're not able to accommodate a class in your current schedule, buy or rent a cookbook filled with nutrient-dense recipes. Many wonderful cookbooks are available to help you learn how to make meals with impact.

Let Water Be Your Main Drink

What helps you prevent headaches, relieve fatigue, maintain a healthy weight, flush toxins, and more? Pure, simple water. Keeping hydrated with water is a simple self-care practice you can do every day. Like its color, it will help keep your mind clear. Water is my drink of choice. Wherever I go, my water bottle (sometimes two) comes along.

The standard eight 8-ounce glasses of water may not be exactly what you need. Your activity level, the weather (if it's super hot and humid outside, you'll naturally be thirsty), whether you're pregnant or breastfeeding, and other factors will determine whether you need more or less water.

You can overdo it. How do you know you're drinking the right amount for you? Look in the toilet after you pee for color and volume. If it is slightly yellow, that generally signals you're hydrated. If it's deep yellow and there is a small amount, it may mean you need to drink more water. If it's totally clear, you're likely drinking too much water.

45 *Write about it: How much water do you drink in a week?*

Purchase a reusable water bottle (many fun, colorful options are available) and note how many ounces it can hold. Keep track of how many times you fill it up throughout the day for one week. At the end of each day, note how you feel related to the amount of water you drank.

46 *Practice it: A wellness elixir: hot water with lemon*

Amp up your water routine by starting your day with room temperature or warm lemon water. Lemon water can help with digestion and detoxification and can boost your immune system. If you don't love lemon, add some sparkle to your glass with oranges, cucumbers, or mint.

Nurture Yourself the Same Way You Nurture Your Children

Before I started my own family, I was not completely connected to what it meant to nurture something fully. The instant I became pregnant, the nurturing flowed. I wanted to take amazing care of myself by eating well and making sure I was getting extra sleep. During my first pregnancy, I would come home from work, take a nap, lead a yoga class, eat dinner, and then go right back to sleep. This was the beginning of my nurturing years. In nurturing my growing baby, I was learning how to nurture myself.

By far, the sweetest, most nurturing moments in my life have been breastfeeding my babies. They would snuggle right up onto my chest as if I were wearing them on my heart. I breastfed my children for a collective two-and-a-half years. That is thousands of ounces of milk and an unlimited amount of nurturing! Throughout those years of breastfeeding, I strengthened my commitment to deeply loving and nurturing myself and giving gratitude to my body. I took more yoga classes, meditated more frequently, and took naps when needed.

As a mama, you are the ultimate nurturer of your children and yourself. Think about how you nurture your children—perhaps you are extra gentle and compassionate with them when they don't follow your rules, or you give them a bath every night so they can sink into a deep, relaxing sleep. Do you nurture yourself the same way? You can mother yourself just as you mother and nurture your children. Mothering yourself is the ultimate manifestation of self-care.

47 *Write about it: How do you nurture?*

Nurturing yourself involves knowing exactly what you need in each moment—a hug, a nap, a quiet space to think. Create a table with two columns. In the left-hand column, list the ways you nurture your children. In the right-hand column, list the ways you nurture yourself. Are your lists balanced? If not, what can you do to honor your need for more nurturing?

48 *Practice it: Abhyanga (self-massage with warm oil)*

One of my all-time favorite self-care practices, the Ayurvedic practice abhyanga, is a luxurious way to nurture yourself. Before a shower or bath, lather on warm coconut oil or sesame oil (as long as you are not allergic to coconut or sesame), beginning at your feet and moving upward toward your heart. Be sure to massage the oil into your shoulders, neck, ears, and head, too. Massage your body lovingly for five to 10 minutes, and then let your skin absorb the oil for at least 10 minutes.

Focus on circular motions at your joints and longer strokes on your arms and legs. Saturating your body with the warm oil is like saturating your body with pure love.

Abhyanga is traditionally practiced in the morning, but I've found that I feel more grounded and fall asleep more easily when I practice it in the evening before bed. Try both and see what works for you. I apply the oil before a shower or bath so my sheets and clothes don't get stained and smell like sesame oil. Keep special towels for your abhyanga practice since they will get oily. Be careful—oil is slippery!

Please note that it is not recommended to practice abhyanga during your menstrual cycle, when you're pregnant, when you have a cold or flu, or with certain medical conditions.

Energize with Balanced Exercise

When you make exercise a habit, your body and mind will endlessly thank you. Among its long list of benefits, exercise helps boost your mood and metabolism and reduces stress. I exercise almost daily for these reasons. Every week, I mix up my exercise routine—some days I attend a yoga class, while other days I pop in a high-intensity fitness DVD or walk outdoors. My goal with exercise is to move my body in ways that feel amazing.

49 *Write about it: Get going with exercise*

The beauty of exercise is that there are many options. How do you feel about exercise? List the types of exercise you enjoy. Then list one exercise you want to try. Can you create space for it this week?

50 *Practice it: Utkatasana (Chair Pose)*

This stimulating pose will energize and rejuvenate you.

- Stand with your inner big toes touching and allow a slice of space in between your heels. Bend your knees and sink your sit bones toward the ground, making sure your knees don't go forward of your toes.

- Extend your arms alongside your ears shoulder-distance apart. Allow your palms to face.

- Take a few breaths. With every exhale, sink your sit bones deeper toward the ground.

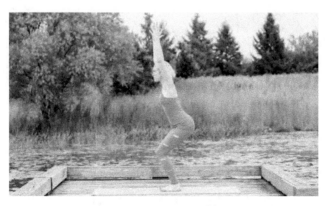

Utkatasana (Chair Pose)

Savor Time Outside

As a child, I spent a lot of my time outdoors in every season—exploring different parks, rollerblading, riding my bike, swimming, ice skating, and sledding. Being with nature feels good—a cool breeze through my hair on a boat ride and the radiant sun on my skin (with sunscreen on) while reading a book near the ocean. As an adult, most of my hours are logged indoors, tending to my to-do list, especially when the weather is not giving me a reason to leave the cozy comfort of my home or office.

Knowing that time in nature is invigorating—it can improve your mood, increase your energy, and decrease anxiety and depression—I look for excuses to go outdoors. My family and I go on long walks, to the park, and we occasionally eat a meal outside.

51 *Write about it: Are you friends with nature?*

Do you devote time to the outdoors every day? List three ways you can spend more time outside this week.

52 *Practice it: Vrksasana (Tree Pose)*

Practice Tree Pose barefoot in the grass or on the ground to feel ultra-connected to Mother Earth.

- Stand with your feet hip-distance apart.

- Root your weight into your left foot as you draw the sole of your right foot to the inside of your left leg—above or below your left knee to protect your knee. If you're building balance, place the toes of your right foot on the ground and your right heel on the inside of your left ankle.

- Press your hands together at your heart or extend your arms above your head with your palms facing. Softly gaze at a point on the ground a few feet in front of you and breathe here for a few moments.

- Imagine your standing foot is the roots of a tree, and ground your roots in self-care. Imagine your body is the trunk, your arms are branches, and your fingers are leaves on a tree. It's OK if you sway—trees sway. Trees also come in different shapes, sizes, and ages.

- Release your right foot to the ground. Repeat on the other side.

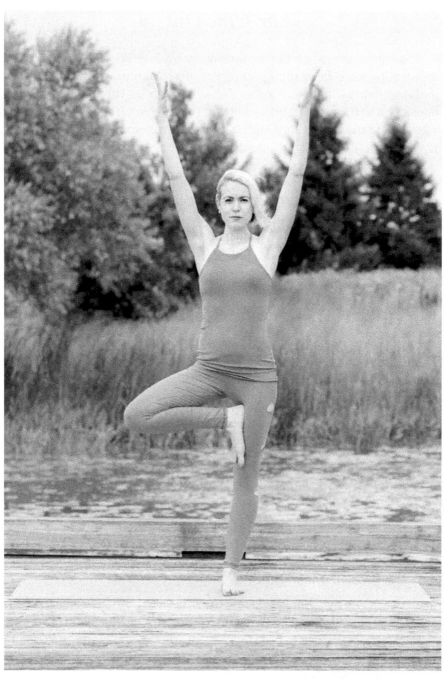

Vrksasana (Tree Pose)

Keep It Clean

I have extensively researched the harmful, cumulative effects of endocrine-disrupting chemicals found in food, beauty products, and household cleaning supplies. Endocrine-disruptors, such as pesticides, phthalates, parabens, and Bisphenol A (BPA), can mimic hormones your body naturally produces or interfere with how hormones function.[2] Scary stuff!

Eating a conventional apple or applying a lipstick with questionable ingredients once in a while isn't as big of a concern as the daily accumulation of eating foods sprayed with harmful pesticides and using products with endocrine-disrupting chemicals. It's the foods you eat, beauty products you use, and what you clean your house with persistently and consistently that can impact your health over time.

Little by little, I began to throw away and stop purchasing products that had ingredients I couldn't pronounce or that are known to be toxic. It was easy to make the switch to healthier cleaning supplies right away. Vinegar and baking soda are cleaning mainstays in my home. I really had to search for beauty products, such as makeup, shampoo, and deodorant, that didn't contain harmful ingredients. Your skin is your body's largest organ, and it absorbs everything you put on it, so it's important to make sure the products you apply are safe to use. Fortunately, there is a larger selection of options today than when I first set out to find healthier personal care items.

Eating as organically as possible was another important switch I made in an effort to live clean. Now, I can taste the difference between an organic strawberry and a conventional strawberry.

It's not realistic to eliminate every chemical you come across, but it's important to reduce your overall exposure. The Environmental Working Group's (EWG's) website (www.ewg.org) is an excellent resource that will help educate you on ways to keep endocrine disruptors out of your life. The EWG posts the annual Shopper's Guide to Pesticides in Produce™ on its website. One of its lists, called the Clean Fifteen, includes foods that you do not need to buy organic, such as avocados and onions, because they aren't as heavily sprayed with pesticides. The other list, called the Dirty Dozen, includes foods you should not eat unless they are organic, such as strawberries and spinach, because they are more heavily sprayed with pesticides.

What does living clean have to do with self-care? Reducing your exposure to harmful chemicals in the foods you eat, beauty products you apply, and household cleaning supplies you use plays a part in keeping you healthy. I'm always discovering new ways to live clean because it's fun! For example, I now practice yoga on an eco-friendly mat.

53 *Write about it: Step one of clean living*

Look at the labels on your beauty products, food, and household cleaning supplies. What is one item in your house from each category that you can eliminate today and replace with a healthier option to help you live clean?

54 *Practice it: Use a tongue scraper*

As with oil pulling, the Ayurvedic practice of cleaning your tongue with a tongue scraper is an oral health superstar. It's a quick, inexpensive practice with a lot of value. (You can buy a plastic tongue scraper from your local grocery store.) Scraping your tongue can help stimulate digestion, enhance your taste, remove plaque and bacteria, and freshen your breath. I practice tongue scraping every morning before oil pulling and brushing my teeth.

- Open your mouth wide, and gently (key word here!) scrape the back of your tongue, pulling the tongue scraper forward to the tip of your tongue.

- Continue to gently scrape your tongue up to five times. Rinse the tongue scraper with clean water after each scrape. Notice any color or residue and the amount.

Get Organized

Take an extra step to live clean by looking at other areas of your life with a fresh perspective—your living space, your work space, your email, and your smartphone. Part of my clean living journey involves decluttering my home, office, and email regularly. This helps clear my mind and gives me a sense of spaciousness.

55 *Write about it: Declutter to make space for more self-care*

Spend time evaluating the items in the room you are sitting in right now. List three things you can easily donate, recycle, or throw away. Tomorrow, pick another room and do the same thing. Keep going until you feel the lightness of decluttering.

56 *Practice it: Viloma Pranayama*

Try this breathing exercise when your mind feels cluttered. Imagine your torso is divided into three sections, which will help you visualize your breath in this practice.

- Begin in a comfortable seated position. Take a full inhale and exhale. Take another deep inhalation and then pause at the top. Slowly exhale a third of the way. Pause. Exhale another third of the way. Pause. Exhale another third of the way, emptying your lungs.

- Inhale smoothly and completely, and repeat the cycle five more times. Then return to your natural breath.

Be Your Own Best Advocate

There have been times in my life where I have allowed others to push me around so much that I lost my voice and the ability to make decisions for myself. When it comes to my health, I draw the line. It has taken years to learn how to become an advocate for my health, but I've finally got it.

I have been taking a low dose of a thyroid medication for about a decade for subclinical hypothyroidism. Hypothyroidism is an underactive thyroid, which means my thyroid gland (the body's master metabolism gland) does not produce enough thyroid-stimulating hormone. This can lead to sluggishness, brain fog, weight gain, and more when not treated.

Over the years, I have combed through research on my symptoms, my treatment options, and how to live well with hypothyroidism. When I was originally diagnosed, I was told that I would need to take medication daily for the rest of my life. Knowing that medications have side effects, I am determined to find more natural ways to treat my hypothyroidism long-term.

Managing stress, going to bed early, getting plenty of sleep, and not overworking myself can impact my thyroid function. Although there are no guarantees that I will be able to stop taking medication for hypothyroidism, this process continues to unfold. As a result, my ability to *speak up* for my wellness has been strengthened. (Interesting, since the butterfly-shaped thyroid gland is located below the voice box.)

57 *Write about it: Do you speak up for yourself?*

Describe ways that you are not being an advocate for yourself and how you can become your own best advocate.

58 *Practice it: Wellness warrior goddess series*

The following is a set of three poses to empower your inner wellness warrior goddess. Practice this series regularly for more confidence and the courage to become your own best advocate.

Virabhadrasana I (Warrior I Pose)

- Stand with your feet hip-distance apart and step your left leg back about three feet. Turn your left foot so that it is planted into the ground at a 45-degree angle. Align the heel of your right foot with the heel of your left foot.

- Keep your left leg straight as you bend your right knee, stacking it over your right ankle. Allow both hips to face forward in the direction of your right foot.

- Sweep your arms overhead and allow your palms to face. Look toward your hands or gaze in front of you.

- Stay here for three breaths. Repeat on the other side.

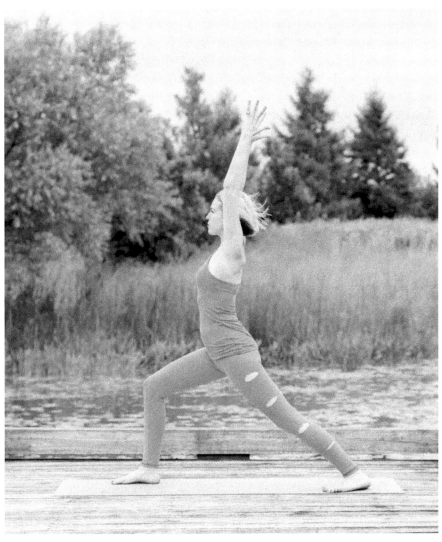

Virabhadrasana I (Warrior I Pose)

Virabhadrasana II (Warrior II Pose)

- Stand with your feet hip-distance apart and step your left leg back about four feet. Turn your left foot in slightly.

- Align the heel of your right foot with the arch of your left foot. Keep your left leg straight as you bend your right knee so it stacks over your right ankle.

- Take your arms to a "T" position with your palms facing down. Relax your shoulders. Spread your fingers wide and gaze toward your right middle finger.

- Stay here for three breaths. Repeat on the other side.

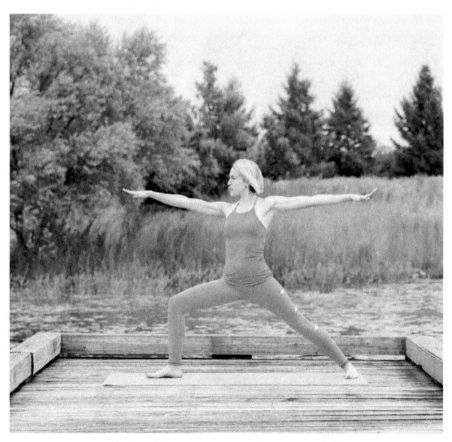

Virabhadrasana II (Warrior II Pose)

Virabhadrasana III (Warrior III Pose)

- Stand with your feet hip-distance apart. Root your right foot into the earth as you launch your left leg off the ground and behind you. Keep your back leg lifted and allow both hips to face the ground.

- As your back leg stays lifted, activate your left foot by flexing your ankle, and bring your hands together at your heart. Glide your torso forward so it is in line with your back leg.

- Gaze at a non-moving object (called your *drishti*) several inches in front of you to help with balance and focus.

- Stay here for three breaths. Repeat on the other side.

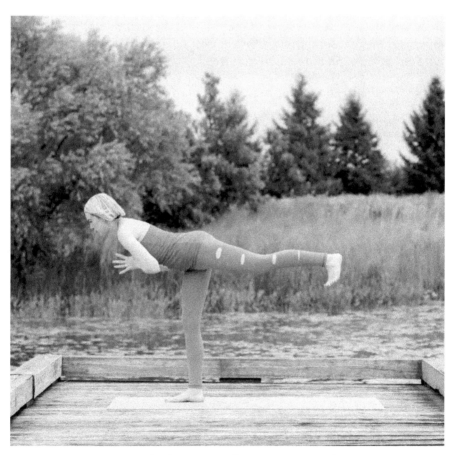

Virabhadrasana III (Warrior III Pose)

Grow Your Gratitude

Thank. You. These two simple words have a profound impact on how you live your life and interact with others. They're words you teach your children to show their appreciation. When you live in gratitude for the abundance in your life, even the little things, such as a compliment someone gave you or a hug from your child, can magnify your gratitude. Emphasizing gratitude—even when your kids won't go to bed, when you're rushing to an appointment, or when you don't get the news you were hoping for—will allow you to appreciate what you already have.

59 *Write about it: 30 days of gratitude*

Every morning when you wake up for the next month, write down one thing you are grateful for in your life. Choose the first thing that comes to mind, but make it something different every day. At the end of the month, note any trends and notice how you feel.

60 *Practice it: Baddha Konasana (Bound Angle Pose)*

Give gratitude to yourself with this pose.

- Begin seated on the ground with your knees bent to either side and the soles of your feet together. Interlace your fingers and place them under your feet.
- Inhale to lengthen your spine, and on an exhale, fold forward over your lower body, allowing your elbows to bend.
- Take a few deep breaths, turning your attention inward.

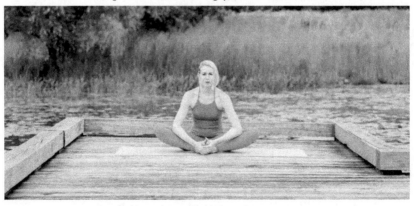

Baddha Konasana (Bound Angle Pose)

Squash Stress and Anxiety

About 40 million adults in the U.S. live with an anxiety disorder, and about half of those living with depression are also living with an anxiety disorder.[3] The self-care practices in this book can help you manage day-to-day anxiety and stress by giving you a renewed outlook on life, but it's important to speak with your doctor if you are concerned about anxiety and depression. Your doctor can recommend a treatment plan for you. There is help. You do not have to quietly suffer.

The life of a modern mama includes dealing with day-to-day stress and the unexpected—reasons to take extra good care of yourself.

I have experienced anxiety—sometimes intense episodes—on and off throughout my life. My level of stress soared to new heights when I became a working mama and placed pressure on myself to do it all. I knew I needed to make a change when I made it a habit to work on my computer, answer text messages, and eat dinner while breastfeeding my baby—talk about multitasking!

Practicing self-care, especially yoga and meditation, has helped me cope with worry and fear so that I am no longer controlled by them.

61 *Write about it: You and stress: How do you deal?*

Think about a stressful moment you experienced recently and describe how you reacted to it. If you could redo that moment, what would you do differently?

62 *Practice it: Nadi Shodhana (Alternate Nostril Breathing)*

Your breath has a profound impact on how you deal with stress and anxiety. Bring balance to both sides of your brain, quiet your mind, and connect to instant relaxation with this centering breathing exercise. This is my go-to practice when I am on edge and need more mental clarity. I like it so much that I have been practicing it every morning.

- Begin in a comfortable seated position.

- Allow your spine to be tall and long. Relax your shoulders. Gently close your eyes. Place your left hand on your left knee with your palm facing down to help ground you.

- Tuck the index and middle fingers of your right hand toward your right palm. Close off your right nostril with your right thumb. Keep that nostril closed as you inhale through your left nostril.

- At the end of the inhale, close off your left nostril with your right ring finger as you simultaneously release your right thumb from your right nostril and exhale out of your right nostril.

- Inhale through your right nostril, close it off using your right thumb, and then release your right ring finger from your left nostril as you exhale through that nostril. Repeat this cycle for a few moments.

- When you're ready, complete this breathing exercise with an exhalation through your left nostril, and then place your right hand on your right knee.

- Take a few cleansing breaths. Guide your attention back to the present moment. Notice the quality of your thoughts. Gently open your eyes.

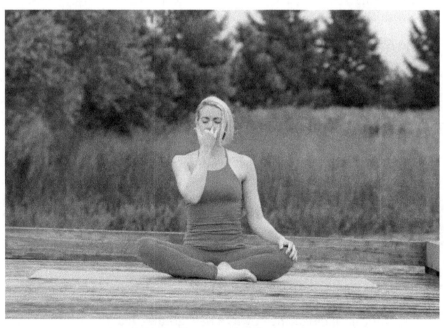

Nadi Shodhana (Alternate Nostril Breathing)

Be the Queen of Compassion

What is your internal dialogue like? Do you judge and criticize yourself, or do you speak delicately to yourself as if you were speaking to a newborn with patience, love, and kindness?

When I shifted my inner voice to be more gentle and positive, I learned how to become my own best friend. Practicing self-compassion allows me to be more compassionate with my husband, my children, coworkers, yoga students, and really anyone I encounter.

One of the most amazing things about practicing compassion is that it helps you realize you are connected to everyone—you have strengths and weaknesses, successes and failures, just as everyone else does.

63 *Write about it: Your inner voice*

Write about your most recent example of negative self-talk, such as criticizing yourself for missing a deadline or for eating something you told yourself you wouldn't eat. How can you replace those thoughts with more positive thoughts?

64 *Practice it: Metta meditation (loving-kindness meditation)*

Metta meditation helps build loving-kindness for yourself and others. This meditation helps expand my compassion more than any other practice. It is so effective that I practice it twice a day. Sending loving, kind thoughts and positive energy to yourself and others is more than just positive vibes. It helps deepen your self-care and your care for others.

This meditation can be practiced in a quiet space in the morning, before starting your workday, just before bed, or with your kids. It will remind you that we all want the same things: happiness, health, peace, and love.

Relax your shoulders. Release any tension in your face and body. Close your eyes or keep them open with a soft gaze. Focus on your breath—smooth, steady breaths in through the nose and out.

Once you have observed your breath for a few moments, repeat the following phrases to yourself quietly or out loud.

For you:

> May I be happy.
> May I be peaceful and at ease.
> May I be well.

Repeat the same phrases with a loved one in mind, substituting "I" with his or her name.

> May _____ be happy.
> May _____ be peaceful and at ease.
> May _____ be well.

Then repeat the phrases with a stranger in mind that you encountered recently.

> May _____ be happy.
> May _____ be peaceful and at ease.
> May _____ be well.

Finally, repeat the phrases with someone you don't get along with.

> May _____ be happy.
> May _____ be peaceful and at ease.
> May _____ be well.

Invest in Your Relationships

You picked up this book, so you already want to be healthier and happier, and to live longer. One way to do all three involves other people—your partner, your kids, your friends, and other important people in your life. The people you most often laugh with, relax with, and enjoy life with can help you live well. Staying connected and involved with people you care about and who care about you is a form of self-care.[4]

Since your social support network is linked to better health,[5] acknowledge whether your current relationships are positive or if they need tweaking. If they require work, think of ways you can make them more enjoyable.

For example, if you're consistently walking away from situations with anger or resentment, try a different approach. Start by checking in with yourself to see if your basic needs are being met. Your toddler might be screaming at the top of her lungs because she doesn't want to take a nap and you just want to rest because you haven't had a day off all week, but identify ways you can make this interaction better. Can you practice more love and compassion with yourself and with her?

65 *Write about it: Who do you like to spend time with most?*

Who makes your heart sing? Write their names and list the attributes you like most about them. Then list how you can spend more time with each person on your list.

66 *Practice it: Date those you love*

Whether it's a date with your partner, your family, or your best friend, schedule one night (or day) each week over the next month to have a date with that person or group. After you come back from your date and you have some quiet time, reflect on what you enjoyed about your date. You get to choose who you spend your time with on this earth. Choose wisely.

Forgive Yourself (and Everyone Else)

I grew up being exceptionally hard on myself, upset when I would get a "B" on a test or when I would make a mistake. It took a lot of emotional energy to maintain the standards I had set for myself. I am happy to report that I have traveled far from this way of thinking. For example, if I forget to do something minor, such as forgetting to run the dishwasher, instead of being harsh with myself, I think, *That's OK. No big deal. I'll remember next time.*

Forgiveness leads to freedom. I come back to the self-care practices in this book to remind myself that I can live with the freedom of forgiveness by transforming negative emotions and thoughts.

Once you forgive yourself, it is easier to forgive others, such as when your husband goes shopping and forgets to buy diapers (for the third week in a row!) even though you wrote him a list and texted him as a reminder.

67 *Write about it: A forgiveness note*

How have you been hurt (or hurt yourself)? What would make it better? Write about it in a letter, and then rip it to pieces as a symbol of forgiveness and moving on.

68 *Practice it: Trikonasana (Triangle Pose)*

Triangle Pose allows space for you to be tender with yourself. Feel freer, lighter, and brighter in less than two minutes.

- Stand with your feet hip-distance apart and step your left leg back about four feet. Turn your left foot in slightly. Line up the heel of your right foot with the arch of your left foot. Keep both legs straight.

- Extend your arms in a "T" position with palms facing down. Inhale to lengthen your spine. On an exhale, reach your right arm toward your right and rest it on your right shin.

- Take your left arm to a 12 o'clock position or place your left hand on your left hip. Stack your left shoulder directly over your right shoulder. Look up toward your left hand or gaze toward your right foot.

- Stay here for three breaths. Repeat on the other side.

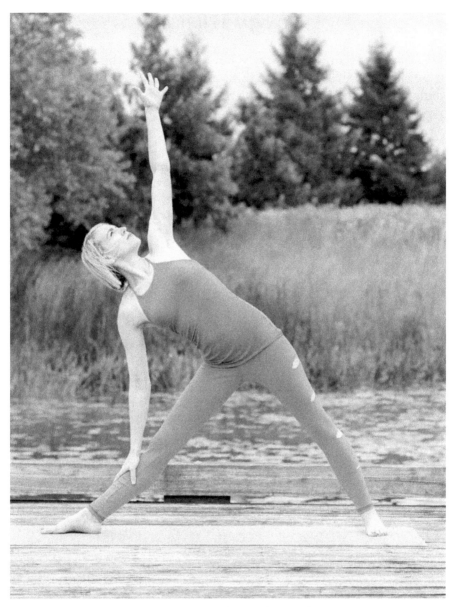

Trikonasana (Triangle Pose)

Accept What Is

Daily life as a mama means you're constantly on the move with few opportunities to rest. (It is often this way for me, too.) Knowing that everything in life is temporary—your job, your toddler's sleep regression, the car you drive, even your house—and that nothing is permanent can breathe new life into your current circumstances.

When your days are filled with people and things shouting at you for attention, practice finding acceptance in the present moment by taking a deep breath and surrendering to what is. Meet yourself where you are.

69 *Write about it: Find acceptance by surrendering*

What do you need to accept and surrender to in this phase of your life?

70 *Practice it: Setu Bandha Sarvangasana (Bridge Pose)*

Surrender to the moment, and find strength in stillness in this pose.

- Begin on your back with knees bent and feet rooted into the ground. Walk your heels toward your sit bones. Rest your arms alongside your body with your palms touching the ground.

- Keep the back of your head on the ground and push through your heels to lift your hips and pelvis toward the sky.

- Stay here, or tuck each shoulder under; interlace your fingers.

- Feel expansion in your collarbone and chest as you send three nourishing breaths to your heart and throat.

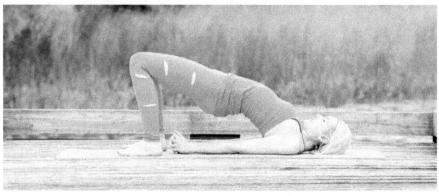

Setu Bandha Sarvangasana (Bridge Pose)

Have Fun with Your Favorites

Yoga, dark chocolate with sea salt, exercising outside—there are certain things I can't live without because they make life brighter and more exciting. When I notice that my mood needs a boost, I recruit one of my favorites to give me a jolt of joy.

71 *Write about it: Make a favorites list and check it twice*

List your favorite

- exercise;
- way to energize;
- self-care practice;
- place to visit;
- book;
- song;
- movie;
- food;
- restaurant;
- store; and
- people.

Review your list and note what makes these your favorites. Visit this list from time to time to evaluate whether your favorites have evolved.

72 *Practice it: Your favorites in one day*

From the list you created, plan something you can look forward to—a date night, a day off, or a weekend getaway that incorporates as many of the items on your list as possible. This mini break from the daily grind generates excitement and can give you a renewed perspective on your life as a very busy mama.

Laugh Loudly and Often

Can you literally laugh your way to wellness? Science says yes. Laughter helps decrease stress, improve your mood, relieve pain, and increase the feel-good chemicals called endorphins that are released by your brain.[6] How does a busy mama with a family to raise fit in more laughter to get the benefits? When your kids are laughing in delight at something funny, join them. When you receive a funny email or text, laugh out loud heartily. Appreciate the lightness that laughter brings.

73 *Write about it: From SOS to LOL*

Do you laugh at yourself and live with a light heart, or do you take life too seriously? Write about your relationship with laughter and whether you get enough of it.

74 *Practice it: Get a daily dose of laughter*

You already know how to laugh, so give yourself more opportunities to do it.

- Laugh away stress with laughter yoga. Search for laughter yoga videos online.
- Watch a comedy or attend a live comedy show.
- Listen to a funny podcast.
- Watch an old home video.
- Spend time with someone who makes you laugh.
- Remember to smile big and often.

Honor the Power of Positivity

"Be the change you wish to see in the world."
— Mahatma Gandhi

Children need positivity in their environment, and that positivity starts with you. You have great influence on your children—the next generation—and your family members, friends, and coworkers just by how you are and the way you interact with them. The best way to teach positivity is to model it. As a mama, you are a natural leader, and you can help lead positive change by beginning to make more positive adjustments in your own life.

Samskaras, or habitual patterns (such as going to bed too late every night), can be challenging to change. You may have a samskara or two that you need to overcome to take the next step in your life. Replacing a negative habit with something positive takes time, effort, practice, and patience. The first step to transforming a samskara is to become aware of it.

A *mantra*—an intention, sacred word, or phrase that is meaningful to you—is essentially a positive affirmation to help you become more aware of negative patterns so that they can be replaced with positive ones. Repeated during *japa* (or mantra meditation), a mantra is traditionally practiced with a string of 108 mala beads plus one guru bead, which is the largest bead on the mala.

Malas are created with beads, stones, and crystals. You can choose one that is meaningful to you based on what you are trying to manifest. For example, if you would like to bring more unconditional love, compassion, peace, and positivity into your life, practice mantra meditation with a rose quartz mala.

75 *Write about it: Your personalized mantra*

Write down a mantra that resonates with you and explore how you can build positive energy, invite it in, channel it, and then set an example for the people in your life.

These are some examples of mantras I use. Choose one that speaks to you or create your own based on the intention you set at the beginning of this book.

I am love.
I am enough.
I am intuitive.
I am creative.
I am compassionate.
I am kind.
I am capable.
I am.

76 *Practice it: Manifest your mantra with mala beads*

To use the mala beads during mantra meditation, hold the mala in one hand. With your other hand, touch the first small bead to the right of the guru bead with your thumb and middle finger of the same hand. Repeat your mantra in your mind or out loud as you touch each bead until you reach the guru bead.

Take your time. Notice the vibration of your mantra and the sensations it creates in your mind, body, and soul.

If you don't have a mala, you can still practice mantra meditation by using your breath as a guide. Practice this basic mantra meditation to connect to your mantra.

- Begin in a comfortable seated position. Allow your spine to be tall and long. Relax your shoulders, and rest your hands on your knees. Gently close your eyes.

- Observe your breath. Each time you inhale, think of the words "I am," and each time you exhale, think of the words "love." Inhale: "I am." Exhale: "love."

- After a few moments of repeating the mantra using your breath, guide yourself back to your natural breath. Open your eyes, and notice how you feel.

Listen Within

Typical daily life does not offer many opportunities to listen to what my body needs. I'm so busy thinking about work and my kids that it is very easy to forget about myself. When I create space to do a quiet activity like journaling, it serves as a reminder that I need to listen more. I notice that when I give myself this quiet time, I am better able to calm the chaos of my external world so my internal world has time to absorb, process, and reflect on what I need.

77 *Write about it: When you don't listen to yourself*

Write about a time when you didn't listen within. Were there consequences of not listening? How did it make you feel?

78 *Practice it: Soak in silence*

If you're used to continuously moving quickly from one task to the next, it's probably challenging for you to sit in silence and listen to what comes up. Plan a time every day—even if it's only for 10 minutes at the end of your day—when you can get out of a noisy environment and have zero interruptions. Choose an activity that doesn't require you to talk, such as drawing or journaling, and allow your soul to speak to you in the silent space. Be receptive, and notice your thoughts and emotions.

Practice Patience

I'm going to start by taking a deep breath.

Motherhood brings patience to a new level, and being a working mama raising little ones has taken my patience to heights I have never seen. Let me give you an example.

When I'm feeling pressed for time, I find myself rushing my son, who I take to preschool in the morning before work. He likes to take his time. He doesn't have meetings to attend or deadlines to meet. If it snows, he will pick up a ball of snow and study it. He'll feel the cold through his mittens and notice that the snow slowly melts the longer he holds it. In the summer, he will find the tiniest ant hill in a crack in the driveway, see ants crawling in and out of their home, and say, "Mama, look at the baby ants. They're so cute!" Meanwhile, I sometimes find myself responding, "Hurry up. Come on. Let's go," trying to get him to sit in his car seat faster.

What message does this send him? That his observations aren't important or that I don't have the time to notice the little things that make his world big and exciting? Although my son tests my patience the most, I learn the most about patience from him. He notices the most minor details and is never in a hurry. When I'm trying to get somewhere on time, I don't always see it his way.

These miniature moments in life are beautiful stopping points that allow time for reflection on what really matters—the little things that my son notices and that I often graze past. If you are constantly whizzing through your day, you too are missing out on a lot of beauty and the opportunity to practice patience.

I get that it's hard to maintain your patience when your kids are taking their time or not listening, but these are the very interactions that are needed to allow your patience to blossom.

It's challenging to be patient when you're not sleeping well, not eating well, not exercising, you have piles of dishes to wash, or you're trying to meet a deadline. These are all reasons why practicing self-care is even more essential to your life.

79 *Write about it: Your breaking point*

Identify the situations in your life when you are most impatient. Is it waiting for people or waiting for something to happen, such as losing weight or getting a new job? Reflect on how you can shift your impatience to patience in these scenarios the next time the opportunity arises.

80 *Practice it: Janu Sirsasana (Head-to-Knee Forward Bend)*

Build patience over time with this pose.

- Begin seated on the ground with your legs extended. Bend your left knee and place the sole of your left foot on the inside of your right inner thigh. Flex your right ankle.

- Inhale to lengthen your spine and sweep your arms up overhead with your palms facing. On an exhale, melt your upper body over your right leg. Allow your hands to touch your shin, ankle, or foot.

- Inhale again to lengthen your spine. Exhale to sink a little deeper into the stretch. Over time, your torso will come closer to your leg. This is fertile ground to practice patience with your body.

- Stay here for a few more breaths. Repeat on the other side.

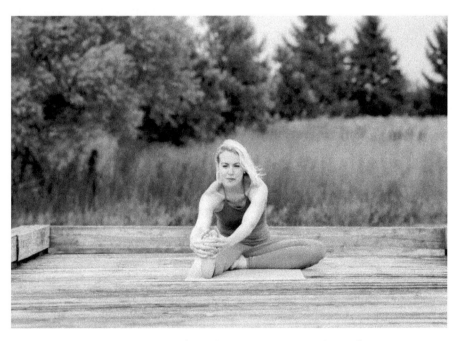

Janu Sirsasana (Head-to-Knee Forward Bend)

Ground Down (First Chakra)

Chakras are invisible, spinning energy fields or vibrations that, when in balance, can help you more easily connect to your highest self and divine truth. You can't see them, but if you observe closely, you can feel if they are out of balance.

Feeling exhausted, overwhelmed, depressed, and anxious are signals that your chakras could use some aligning. Before discovering chakra practices, my brain buzzed with thoughts. One thought would jump so quickly to the next thought, I barely had time to catch up to what I was originally thinking. After bringing balance to my chakras, I felt a noticeable difference in my thoughts, mood, and energy.

The chakra-inspired practices that follow will help restore harmony to your mind, body, and spirit and further lead you down your self-care path. You may have different ideas and interpretations as you practice these. Know that your interpretation is beautiful and unique.

As a working mama, I have a lot going on—multiple and constant thoughts, ideas, and responsibilities. If you do too, you can benefit from the following grounding practice. Your first chakra—the *muladhara chakra,* or root chakra—helps you connect to your basic needs, the earth, and your family, or "roots." When balanced, it helps you feel centered, safe, and grounded.

81 *Write about it: Connect to your roots*

Write about whether you feel connected to your root chakra. Are your basic needs being met? Do you feel secure and grounded?

82 *Practice it: Get grounded meditation*

This meditation brings awareness to your first chakra.

- Sit on the ground or a chair. Allow your spine to be tall and long. Relax your shoulders, and place your palms on your knees. Gently close your eyes.

- Bring your attention to your breath. Watch your inhales and exhales come and go.

- Visualize a bright red light emanating from the base of your spine, the seat of your root chakra. Red is the color associated with this chakra. Notice if the red light is spinning. If it is, is it spinning slowly or quickly?

- Notice if the energy from the red light brings any sensations or warmth to the base of your spine. With each inhale, allow the red light to grow and become so luminous that it fills your entire body.

- Find stillness in this red light and notice what feelings and thoughts are present.

- After a few moments, slowly let the light fade into the space at the base of your spine, and bring your attention back to the present moment. Inhale and exhale deeply through your nose. Gently open your eyes.

Unearth Your Creative Sparkle
(Second Chakra)

I am my most creative self when I don't feel pressured or hurried and when I create space to do the things I love. When I make self-care a priority, I notice my creativity flows more effortlessly more often.

The second chakra—the *svadhisthana chakra* or sacral chakra—is the seat of creativity and connects you with your ability to feel. It's where babies grow and ideas are planted.

83 *Write about it: Unleash innovation*

What do you want to create in your life right now? Write about your creative vision.

84 *Practice it: New creation meditation in Supta Baddha Konasana (Reclining Bound Angle Pose)*

Practice the following meditation to let your creativity flow.

- Begin on your back with your head and shoulders on the ground.

- Bend your knees and allow them to fall to either side as you press the soles of your feet together. If you'd like, place a yoga block, book, or blanket on either side of the outside of your outer thighs or knees for support.

- Place your left hand on your heart and your right hand on your belly below your navel—the location of the sacral chakra. Observe your breath. Notice the rise of your belly and right hand on your inhales, and how your belly and hand recede toward your spine on your exhales.

- Visualize yourself planting a seed in your low belly for something you want to grow. Maybe it's an idea for a project. Maybe it's a baby. Watch this seed sprout, and then visualize its fullest potential. Feel confident that this beautiful creation can be brought to life.

- After a few breaths, bring your attention back to the present moment, and open your eyes.

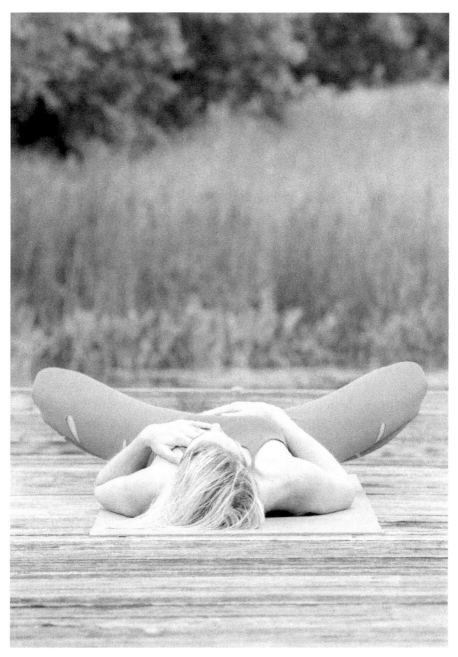

Supta Baddha Konasana (Reclining Bound Angle Pose)

Ignite Your Inner Fire (Third Chakra)

I feel more like a warrior than a worrier when my solar plexus—the *manipura chakra* or navel chakra—is in balance. You can feel bright like the sun—empowered and energetic—by connecting to this chakra.

85 *Write about it: Your power*

Write about a time when you tapped into your personal power, felt like you were fulfilling your life's purpose, or believed in yourself.

86 *Practice it: Navasana (Boat Pose) with Candle Visualization*

Awaken your navel chakra and your abs with this powerful pose.

- Begin seated with your knees bent and feet on the ground. Engage your abdominal muscles as you lift your legs and feet off the ground to a 90-degree angle.

- Allow your arms to extend alongside your legs. Keep your chest lifted as you draw your shoulder blades together.

- Close your eyes and imagine a steady, glowing candle flame at the center of your navel. Notice its intensity and brightness. Is it yellow (the color associated with the navel chakra)? This candle represents your inner fire—the source of your inner power. Tap into this flame by visualizing it whenever you need more drive to move forward.

- After a few more breaths, open your eyes.

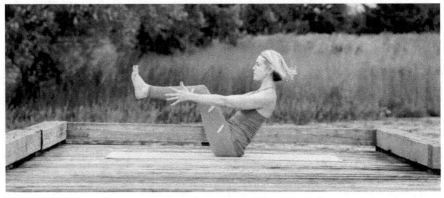

Navasana (Boat Pose)

Give Yourself the Greatest Gift (Fourth Chakra)

When I was 19 years old, I was determined to be perfect. I had goals and nothing was going to get in my way of achieving them. I was an aspiring model and a natural overachiever in school with a flawless GPA and perfect attendance. I was the student who did extra credit when it wasn't necessary. This perfectionist behavior turned into excessively exercising when my exhausted body needed rest and scrutinizing every calorie I consumed when I clearly craved more energy.

For months, I ignored the obvious signals (actually, red alerts) my body gave me. My stomach would growl intensely. I would ignore it. I thought I could train myself to not be hungry.

Because I wasn't completely starving myself, I didn't think any of this was a big deal. But I was intentionally restricting the foods I ate, eating only fruits, vegetables, whole grains, no-fat or low-fat foods, and very little protein. Analyzing and monitoring every bite was something that I could control when everything else felt like it was out of my control.

At one point, I was swimming in size zero jeans and experiencing regular heart palpitations. There were times I felt so faint, lightheaded, and dizzy that when I stood up, I saw stars.

After months of this vicious cycle—depriving myself of calories and exercising too much—I stopped getting my period. That was scary because then I started to question whether this would impact me when I wanted to start a family.

One afternoon, I vividly remember running full speed on my worn-out treadmill. When I tried to cool down, my heartbeat wouldn't regulate. It remained elevated when I went to bed that night, and that's when I became fully aware that something was seriously wrong. I shivered myself to sleep.

That night was a turning point.

I woke up the next morning, desperate to feel better, feel like me again. One day at a time, I began to mother myself back to health. I taught myself how to love myself again, that I was worthy of my own self-love.

Unfortunately, I knew I was not alone in struggling with the overpowering reigns of an eating disorder. About 30 million people in the U.S. are living with an eating disorder.[7] If you are one of them, I want you to know that you deserve to feel better, and there is absolute hope for your full recovery.

Please reach out to your doctor and contact an eating disorder helpline. Find information about support groups on the National Association of Anorexia Nervosa and Associated Disorders website at www.anad.org.

As I reflect on this experience, many things contributed to my undiagnosed eating disorder—my fascination with perfectionism, depriving myself of essential nutrients, the over-exercising, the images I was bombarded with in the media from a very young age, and comments I absorbed from other people.

It took years of fully accepting who I am—mind, body, and spirit—to completely recover from distorted thoughts about food and body image. My journeys with pregnancy and breastfeeding strengthened my self-love. They taught me that my whole self, at every stage in life, deserves to be celebrated and honored.

When I was learning how to take better care of myself, I wrote love notes to my body to let it know it is deserving of kindness, love, and respect. These notes were expressions of opening my *anahata chakra,* or heart chakra.

When your heart chakra is in balance, love, compassion, and forgiveness effortlessly flow. Create the space and time every day for your self-love to bloom.

87 *Write about it: A love letter to you*

What is the most amazing thing about your body? What do you want to tell it? How can you become best friends with your body?

88 *Practice it: Lead with your heart meditation*

The following meditation will help open your heart chakra.

- Begin in a comfortable seated position. Allow your spine to be tall and long. Relax your shoulders. Place your hands on your heart, and gently close your eyes.

- Take a moment to observe your breath. Once your breath is smooth, connect with your heartbeat. Notice it. Feel it. Is it beating rapidly or is it steady? As it beats, give gratitude to it for pumping for you throughout your life—during the calm, peaceful moments, during the stressful moments, and all of the moments in between.

- Think of the one thing you love most about yourself. Let that image or word naturally appear. Know that the rest of you is deserving of this love, too.

- Inhale deeply, and on an exhale, shine and spread a warm, loving light to every inch of your being. Allow yourself to feel cared for, respected, and valued.

- After a few breaths, bring your attention back to the present moment. Open your eyes with a renewed view on self-love. Carry this feeling with you throughout your day and come back to this meditation when you need it.

Be Real. Be Raw. Be You. (Fifth Chakra)

How often do you show the world the real you? Do you feel free to express your true self?

I used to carry around a genuine people-pleasing mentality. Boy, was that a big weight to bear. I thought, if I do things people like, then they won't judge me. This way of living masked my ability to live authentically.

Being more transparent and honest with myself and with others in my thoughts, words, and actions helped me to find my real voice. I did this by bringing balance to the *vishuddha chakra,* or throat chakra, which is located in the throat. A balanced throat chakra can help guide you to your inner truth and authenticity. Now (yes, right now!) is the time to embody your most authentic self so you can start to speak and live your truth.

89 *Write about it: An exercise in authenticity*

Think about a recent situation when you weren't living authentically. Describe what you said and did. Then describe the situation as if you had said and done things from your most authentic self, choosing words and actions that align with who you really are.

90 *Practice it: Speak your truth meditation*

This meditation will help you express yourself and articulate your thoughts, feelings, and needs more clearly.

- Begin in a comfortable seated position. Allow your spine to be tall and long. Relax your shoulders, and rest your hands on your knees. Gently close your eyes.

- Bring your attention to your breath. Deepen your inhales and exhales by making the sound of ocean waves crashing on the shore at the back of your throat with each inhale and exhale.

- Visualize a bright blue light beginning to illuminate your throat. This is the color associated with the throat chakra. Notice if the light is spinning and whether the light's energy brings any sensations or warmth to where it shines.

- Allow the light to grow and become brighter so that it fills your entire body, helping you connect to your authentic inner voice. Feel the light's power in your muscles and bones, penetrating the deepest layers to crack open the real you.

- After a few moments, let the light fade and bring your attention back to the present moment. Inhale and exhale deeply through your nose. Gently open your eyes. Carry authenticity into your day by being honest with yourself and the others in your life.

Trust Yourself (Sixth Chakra)

Have you ever thought about a song and then you turn on the radio and that song is playing? Or have you thought about someone and then seconds later you get a text message or call from that person? These are little glimpses of your intuition.

One example of intuition that stands out in my mind was when I was pregnant with my first child. I predicted that he would arrive earlier than his due date and that he would break my water. That's exactly what happened. He was a vivacious, active little guy in the womb, constantly kicking and punching. A few days before I was 38 weeks pregnant, my water broke. What was most interesting was that it had broken in only one pocket—the space where he delivered the most kicks.

The universe is always serving up signs and signals to help guide you to a deeper connection of inner knowing. Have you awakened enough to fully receive these gifts?

One way to stimulate your intuition is by connecting to your *ajna chakra,* or third-eye chakra, which resides in the space between your eyebrows.

91 *Write about it: Are you intuitive?*

Have you recognized a situation, which was more than just a coincidence, when you intuitively knew something was about to happen? Describe your most intuitive experiences and what they have taught you.

92 *Practice it: Inner wisdom meditation*

This meditation will help you connect to your intuition, insight, and inner wisdom, and guide you to the answers that are already within you.

- Begin in a comfortable seated position. Allow your spine to be tall and long. Relax your shoulders. Gently close your eyes.

- Touch your index fingertips to your thumb tips, extending the other three fingers on each hand. Rest the back of your hands on your knees. This is Gyan Mudra, a mudra to help connect you to knowledge and wisdom.

- Visualize a glowing indigo light between the space of your eyebrows. This is the color associated with the third-eye chakra.

- Notice if the light is spinning and whether it brings any sensations or warmth to that space. As the indigo light begins to expand, allow it to help you see things in your life with more clarity and precision. Trust that this light will help guide you to your intuition and inner wisdom as you move forward in life.

- After a few moments, slowly let the light fade and bring your attention back to the present moment. Inhale and exhale deeply through your nose. Gently open your eyes.

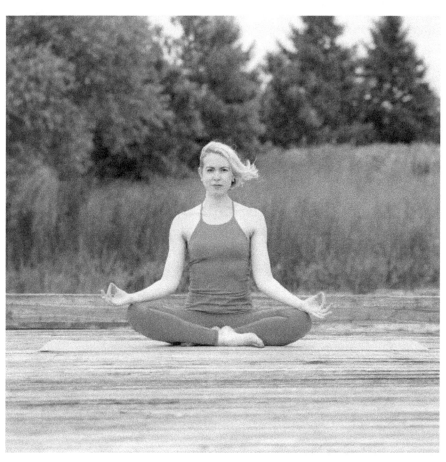

Gyan Mudra

Call Upon Your Highest Self (Seventh Chakra)

One day I was feeling particularly curious about defining my highest self—my most confident, intelligent, calm, peaceful, and wise presence—so I put pen to paper and wrote this manifesto.

I am not anxious or fearful.
I am calm and courageous.

I am not judgmental or critical.
I am accepting and understanding.

I am not angry or impatient.
I am gentle and patient.

I am not invisible or scattered.
I am confident and centered.

I am not competitive or resentful.
I am fair and forgiving.

I am not jealous or negative.
I am satisfied and positive.

My highest self radiates light throughout my being and into the world.

It is pure. It is love. It is truth.

It is an inner knowing that I am connected to everything; everything is connected to me.

It is always watching. Gracefully waiting. Ready to serve. Prepared to inspire.

When in balance, the *sahasrara chakra,* or crown chakra, which is located on the crown of your head, can help you connect to your highest self and divine truth.

93 *Write about it: Your highest self manifesto*

Create your own manifesto as an offering to your highest self.

94 *Practice it: Enlighten your life meditation*

Bring awareness to your crown chakra with this meditation.

- Begin in a comfortable seated position. Allow your spine to be tall and long. Relax your shoulders, and rest your hands on your knees. Gently close your eyes. Bring your attention to your breath.

- Visualize a lotus flower blooming with violet light on the crown of your head. This is the color associated with the crown chakra. Allow the light from each petal to glow as its beams shine toward the sky, offering a deeper connection of your mind, body, and spirit to the universe.

- After a few moments, let the light from the petals fade. Bring your attention back to your breath and the present moment. Gently open your eyes.

Let Go of What No Longer Serves You

"When I let go of what I am,
I become what I might be." —Lao Tzu

This quote reminds me that when I let go of the pressure I place on myself to be everything I am, I am open to becoming everything I might be. As a modern mama, you probably place numerous unnecessary demands on yourself, and you may unknowingly allow others to place stress on you as well. Help set yourself free by letting go of any unrealistic expectations and the need for you to do everything everyone expects you to do.

As I have mentioned, I grew up a rule follower. Throughout school and early on in my 20s, I did what I was told and accommodated requests from others before my own. I tolerated other people's ideas of what I should be doing. I ignored the fact that these demands caused me anxiety.

I had to dig deep with self-inquiry and self-study, but I began to chip away and learn how to let go of other people's unrealistic expectations of me so that I could develop into who I might be.

95 *Write about it: What you need to let go of (and why)*

What are you holding onto that no longer serves you? Why is now the time to let it go?

96 *Practice it: Let it go meditation*

This meditation will help you prepare for letting go of the things in your life that no longer serve you.

- Begin in a comfortable seated position. Allow your spine to be tall and long. Relax your shoulders. Gently close your eyes.

- Place your left hand on your belly and your right hand on top of your left hand. Observe your breath. Watch your inhales and exhales come and go.

- On an inhale, think of something—a thought, a material object, a habit, a relationship—that no longer serves you. On an exhale, mentally let it go. Inhale, think of it again, and then exhale, let it go.

- Repeat this for a few more breaths until you feel that you have fully let go of that which no longer serves you.

- With your breath as your guide, keep letting it go until you feel a sense of lightness. Release yourself from the energy this carried and that you have been holding onto for so long.

- Gently bring your attention back to the present moment. Inhale and exhale deeply through your nose. Open your eyes. You are ready to take action to physically let it go.

Realize You Are Enough

Who I show up as a mama, partner, employee, coworker, and friend is enough, but for years, I didn't believe it. Growing up, success was measured by my ability to perform, accomplish, and achieve. In many ways, I still aim to do these things, but the difference now is that instead of pushing past my limits at the expense of my self-care, I respect what I need first.

This is a revolutionary way of living because many people are praised for striving for more and excelling at the highest level—working extra hours, cooking an organic dinner every night, planning a perfect vacation, and on and on. It has become a badge of honor to tell others that you haven't slept well for weeks because to them that means you're being super productive. What are you trying to prove by doing more?

While I admit this line of thinking has allowed me many opportunities, it limited my self-care. After some exploration, I finally understood the root of why I was always doing more. It resulted from my own feelings of not being enough and that I could/should be doing more—even though I was already doing way more than enough.

It is not sustainable to overwork yourself. It will beat you down. Understandably, there will be periods in your life where you will work more. Caring for young children or meeting a major deadline are some examples, but if you make this a habit, it will show up as anxiety, stress, depression, and a feeling of depletion.

Balance work with rest. Give yourself permission to take incredible care of yourself and know when enough is enough.

97 *Write about it: When enough is enough*

Do you sometimes overwork yourself and do more, even though your body and mind are begging for rest? What are the signals that you've had enough?

98 *Practice it: Mantra meditation: I am enough*

Embrace that you are enough with this simple meditation.

- Begin in a comfortable seated position. Allow your spine to be tall and long. Relax your shoulders, and rest your hands on your knees. Gently close your eyes.

- Observe your breath. Each time you inhale, think of the words "I am," and each time you exhale, think of the words "enough." Inhale: "I am." Exhale: "enough." Embody these words with each breath.

- After a few moments of repeating the mantra using your breath, guide yourself back to the present moment. Open your eyes. Notice how you feel.

Play Every Chance You Have

Have you ever noticed how young children live in the present moment? Their faces light up when they're playing at the park or with their favorite toy. Meanwhile, the only thing that might be keeping you in the present moment is a cup of coffee. There is a major disconnect here. At what point in life do people stop living in the present moment? Is it when they stop playing?

With demands from rushing around, working, and taking care of a family, it's easy to get into the mentality of work, rush, work, repeat, with no time for play. This routine does not inspire spontaneous playfulness. Allow your children to help you rediscover the joy of playing.

99 *Write about it: Channel your inner child*

What activities from childhood can you do now that will rekindle playfulness and joy?

100 *Practice it: Balasana (Child's Pose)*

This playful pose will help spark joy. Practice it with a smile or with your kids.

- Begin on your hands and knees in tabletop position with your shoulders stacked over your wrists, your hips stacked over your knees, and the tops of your feet on the ground.

- Draw your sit bones toward your heels as you extend your arms forward, keeping your palms on the earth. Connect your forehead to the ground. You can rest your belly on your thighs or widen your knees.

- Soften your belly and heart as you breathe into any areas of tension.

- Find playfulness in this pose. You can walk your hands to the right for a few breaths and then to the left.

- When you're ready, walk your hands back to center and return to tabletop position.

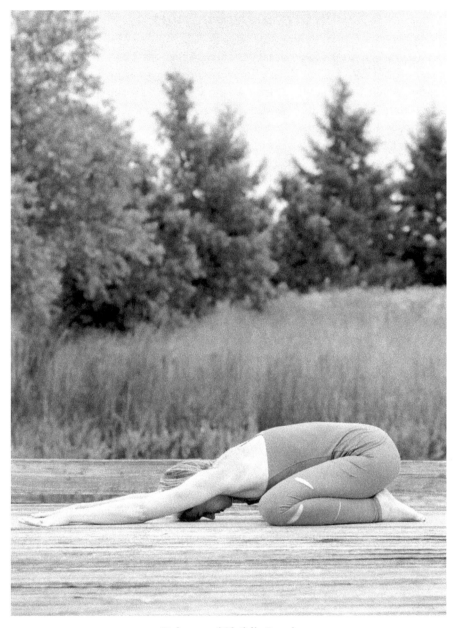

Balasana (Child's Pose)

Start a Daily Journal

In grade school, I kept a diary that had a lock on it and the words "Keep Out" on the cover. That didn't deter my little sister from finding the key, reading what I wrote, and learning who I had a crush on at the time. But I still maintained my diary because I liked recording the day's events in it. Keeping a diary gave me a taste of what it is like to journal.

Journaling is more than a rehashing of your day. When practiced regularly, it is a transformative channel that sparks creativity and helps you focus on and prioritize the things that matter most to you.

This is another one of my all-time favorite self-care practices, which is no surprise to me as I have a journalism degree and I love to write. Journaling is a different type of writing. It's a collection of your thoughts, inspirations, goals, and dreams—writing for your eyes only.

I journaled on and off for several years, and it was when I started to journal every night before bed as part of a yearlong intention that I reconnected with my lifelong goal of publishing the book you are reading now. I realized all the different journals I was writing in—three or more at any given time—had a higher purpose: to inspire me to write this book.

Every page in a journal is a blank canvas, a new opportunity. If you're out of practice or don't know where to start, purchase a journal or book with writing prompts (like this one), or use a simple notebook.

I like to break away from technology when I journal, so I use pen and paper, but you can also type your thoughts or record your voice. Do what works for you.

Tips to get you started:

- Date your entries and occasionally look back to review what you wrote. Notice any topics you write about consistently, and how much you've grown in your writing and your life.

- Write about what inspires and interests you.

- Be honest with yourself. There's no competition and no one to please, so write truthfully and from your heart.

- Allow one thought to flow into the next.

- Keep writing. Make it a habit. Write in the morning before you leave your bedroom or at night before bed.

- Take your journal with you wherever you go. Any time you are inspired by a conversation, a song, a meal, or nature, write down your thoughts right away.

101 *Write about it: How to begin your next journal*

Here's a writing prompt to start your next journal: What did you learn from the writing prompts, yoga poses, and self-care practices in this wellness guide? Which practices resonated with you most? Which practices can you share with other mamas, your friends, and your coworkers?

102 *Practice it: Rejuvenate your mind before you write*

Reinvigorate your mind with this quick practice.

- Begin in a comfortable seated position. Allow your spine to be tall and long. Relax your shoulders. Gently close your eyes.

- Bring your hands together a few inches in front of your heart and rub them back and forth as quickly as possible for several breaths, creating friction.

- Once you have created heat between your palms, cup your palms over your eyes. Keep your palms here for three breaths, calling upon your intuition and clarity of your thoughts to help guide you to express yourself through writing. Uncover your eyes, and with a fresh perspective, begin to write.

Sleep Deep: Your Bedtime Routine

What mama isn't tired? A mom's day is never done—or so it seems because there is always more to do. More than a third of American adults don't get enough sleep,[8] but getting quality sleep consistently is one of the most significant things you can do for your health and wellness. Sleep is not a luxury; it is a necessity because it is restorative to the body. You need sleep like you need water.

If you're a working mama, after you leave work, you move on to part two of your day: picking up kids, dinnertime, bath time, and bedtime—so many to-dos in a short amount of time. Once the kids are in bed and the house is quiet, there is more to do. When you finally have time for yourself, it's likely late. You might find yourself staying up even later to read a book or to scroll through social media posts.

Going to bed is the ultimate act of letting go of your day, but you need to do a little prep to signal your mind and body that it's OK to wind down. Help your body sink into restful slumber so that you can get the sleep you need by creating a consistent bedtime routine, which includes going to bed at the same time every night.

103 *Write about it: Seven-day sleep challenge*

Keep track of your sleep for a week. See if you can dedicate one-third of every day to sleep. Chart the day, time you went to bed, the time you woke up, and your mood upon waking.

At the end of the week, evaluate the consistency of your mood vs. the amount of sleep you had. What tweaks do you still need to make?

104 *Practice it: Viparita Karani (Legs-Up-the-Wall Pose)*

This delicious pose is a real treat. It will help promote restful sleep by unwinding your body and soothing your nervous system, especially if practiced just before bed.

Find an area of the wall where you have space to get in and out of this pose. You can place a folded blanket under your hips.

- Sit close to a wall with the left side of your body next to it and your knees bent. Carefully roll your low back to the ground and rest the back of your head.

- Straighten your legs and move the back of your legs and sit bones toward the wall so they touch it. Flex your ankles, and then rest your arms on the ground in a "T" position, or place one hand on your heart and one hand on your belly.

- Stay in this position for as long as you need.

- When you're ready to come out of it, soften your knees and wiggle your sit bones off the wall as you roll to your left side. Rest here for a moment with your knees curled toward your chest. Push your right palm into the earth, slowly making your way to a comfortable seated position.

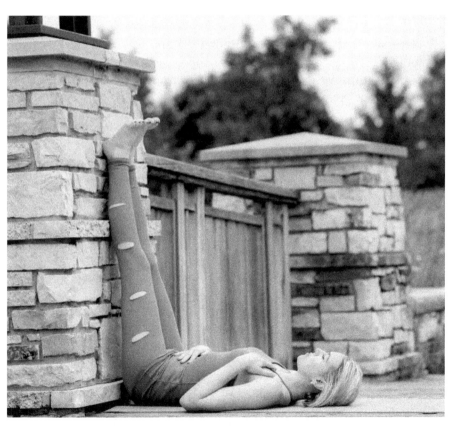

Viparita Karani (Legs-Up-the-Wall Pose)

Just Be

Mamas are human *beings*, not human *doings*, but many of us have become so accustomed to doing everything for everyone that *doing* has become a way of life—it has consumed our lives. The pose below is the ultimate action of non-doing. Practice it often and reap the benefits of just being.

105 *Write about it: Nothing to do, nowhere to be*

Describe how it feels to just be—when you are free of worries and hurried thoughts—similar to how you feel in Savasana.

106 *Practice it: Savasana (Final Relaxation Pose)*

Savasana is traditionally practiced at the end of a yoga class, but you can practice it on its own. In fact, if you only have time to practice one yoga pose, make it this one. Savasana invites you to find peace and stillness in the moment by giving yourself permission to just be. This relaxing practice is a reminder that it's not up to you to be everything to everyone.

- Lie down on your mat or the ground with your legs extended. Allow your ankles and feet to fall away from each other. Bring your arms alongside your body with your palms facing up.

- Let the back side of your body melt like butter into your mat.

- Gently close your eyes and connect with your breath. Thoughts will inevitably pop up, such as *What's for dinner?* or *Did I schedule that appointment?* Acknowledge those thoughts and then gently guide your attention back to your breath.

- Take rest. Stay here for as long as you need. There's nowhere to rush; nowhere to go.

- When you're ready to come out of the pose, gently reawaken your body by slowly touching your thumb tips to each fingertip, and then circle your wrists and ankles.

- Bring your knees toward your chest and wrap your arms around your shins to give yourself a big hug—you deserve it!

- Gently roll to your left-hand side with your knees still bent. Use your left arm as a pillow to support your head as you place your right hand on the earth. Allow your muscles, bones, and organs to rest. After a few moments, push into your right palm and slowly come to a comfortable seated position.

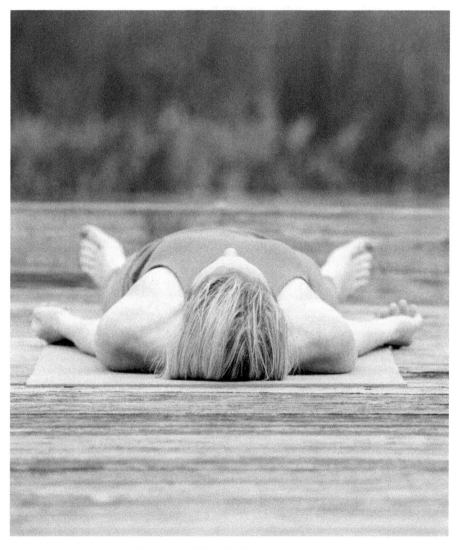

Savasana (Final Relaxation Pose)

Resolve to Stay Committed to Lifelong Self-Care

Congratulations! You have explored and unearthed self-care practices to help your mind, body, and spirit bloom so that your whole being can buzz with wellness. I am proud of you and your dedication to take good care of yourself. As you move through the seasons of the year and the seasons of your life, adjust your wellness practices as needed. Keep learning new ways to take good care of yourself every day.

You've got this, and you are deserving of every ounce of self-care.

107 *Write about it: How to stay motivated on your wellness path*

Write a motivational message to keep your commitment to self-care. Post it where you can see it. Live it. Breathe it. Become it. Let it serve as inspirational fuel for positive transformation.

108 *Practice it: Meditate in front of your vision board and dedication space*

Choose your favorite meditation from this book, and meditate facing your dedication space and vision board to maintain a continuous connection to your intention and self-care.

A Final Wellness Wish for You

Recall the intention you set at the beginning of this book. Take note of what you have learned about yourself along the way. Although you have come to the end of this book, you are not at the end of your self-care journey. Consistently standing up for your self-care is a lifelong practice. It needs to be maintained for you to continue to thrive.

You have the tools to live a centered and vibrant life. I encourage you to refer to the notes you have written and the practices in this book over and over again, and to allow them to serve as a reminder to you that when you give to yourself, you can give so much more to others. You are worth the time and energy it takes to take care of you. Stay inspired by visiting www.juliegtheyogi.com and share your self-care stories on Facebook and Instagram @juliegtheyogi.

As a mama, you have more influence than you will ever know. You have the power to be a wellness leader in your home, at work, and anywhere else life leads you. By taking good care of yourself, you naturally inspire others to do the same. I am excited for you to be the luminous light this world needs. Shine on!

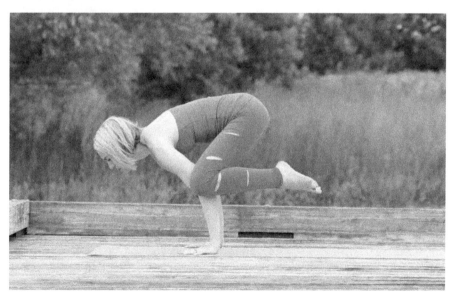

Bakasana (Crow Pose)
Visit www.juliegtheyogi.com to learn how to practice Crow Pose and for more self-care practices and ideas.

References

1. 2016 Yoga in America Study by Yoga Journal and the Yoga Alliance. (2016). Retrieved from www.yogajournal.com/page/yogainamericastudy

2. Endocrine disruptors. National Institute of Environmental Health Sciences. Retrieved from www.niehs.nih.gov/health/materials/endocrine_disruptors_508.pdf

3. Facts and statistics. Anxiety and Depression Association of America. Retrieved from https://adaa.org/about-adaa/press-room/facts-statistics

4. Can relationships boost longevity and well-being? (2017). Harvard Health Letter. Retrieved from www.health.harvard.edu/mental-health/can-relationships-boost-longevity-and-well-being

5. The determinants of health. World Health Organization. Retrieved from www.who.int/hia/evidence/doh/en

6. Stress relief from laughter? It's no joke. Stress management. (2016). Mayo Clinic. Retrieved from www.mayoclinic.org/healthy-lifestyle/stress-management/in-depth/stress-relief/art-20044456

7. Eating disorder statistics. National Association of Anorexia Nervosa and Associated Disorders. Retrieved from www.anad.org/education-and-awareness/about-eating-disorders/eating-disorders-statistics

8. 1 in 3 adults don't get enough sleep. (2016). Centers for Disease Control and Prevention. Retrieved from www.cdc.gov/media/releases/2016/p0215-enough-sleep.html

CPSIA information can be obtained
at www.ICGtesting.com
Printed in the USA
LVHW081927080219
606934LV00009B/26/P

9 781942 891840